Invertebrate Neurons and Behavior

edited by
C. A. G. Wiersma

The MIT Press
Massachusetts Institute of Technology
Cambridge, Massachusetts

INVERTEBRATE NEURONS AND BEHAVIOR

Introduction

C. A. G. WIERSMA

THE FORBIDDING numbers of individual nerve cells that form the central nervous system of all vertebrates and that are usually still formidable, though considerably smaller, in those invertebrates that can be handled by present techniques, have led to the view that single-cell reactions are of little or no value for the analysis of brain function. But, as amply demonstrated in this volume, there are now many examples in both invertebrates and vertebrates of aggregations of cells, in which each member appears to have a circumscribed functional connectivity and mode of reaction. Especially in the invertebrates, a number of such cells can be unambiguously recognized and named, being present in all normal individuals of a given species. Identifiable interneurons on the sensory side are interesting, because their responses indicate which features in the environment are selected as important for the animal. Interneurons on the motor side often illustrate by their patterned output the existence of preprogrammed patterns of muscle contractions. In both cases modulation by other pathways than their main input channel can be studied, considerably enhancing the understanding of how central and local factors are integrated. Such influences are present in the most simple of all behavioral reactions, the monosynaptic reflex, and the study of cases in which input and output are provided by one or more identified neurons will be very rewarding, as indicated by several of the following chapters. Interneurons that are high-level links in complex behavioral reactions are good monitors of the mechanism by which such reactions are obtained, and their study may be expected to provide important insights for correlating neural and behavioral events. Concerning the applicability of these concepts to even more complex nervous systems, it looks at present that although they abide by very similar rules (see especially Bullock in this part), such systems do not have the same extreme degree of predestination. Even when no neuron is quite like any other in a large population of interneurons subserving a given overall function, the differences among neighboring cells might be so small that loss of a number of them would not result in noticeable change in output. In such cases a statistical approach might be the most fruitful methodology. But it should be noted that the underlying principle could be the same, enhancing the value of studying the simpler invertebrate systems.

The different chapters in this part are divided according to the main divisions of the higher invertebrates. There are sound reasons for such a treatment, because even though nervous systems are among the least variable organs in evolution and show pronounced overall similarities, differences, especially important to methods of investigation, are also present. For instance, in molluscs, the presence of peripheral connections that allow reflex activity in the absence of the central ganglia represent difficulties for evoked behavioral responses, especially because it is not yet very clear how these systems interact. The cephalopod molluscs are even more complex in that the number of their central nervous elements is very large (Young, 1971), so that their investigation presents the same type of difficulties as vertebrates and may thus form the same type of hindrance for investigations at the cellular level. On the other hand, they share with vertebrates a very readily established conditioned behavior for various stimuli and are furthermore distinguished by the presence of two memories, one for visual and one for tactile stimuli. Annelids appear to have integration of sensory input at a very early stage (Nicholls and Baylor, 1968), so that sensory fibers entering their central nervous systems become comparable to those of arthropod interneurons, representing large surface areas only. Insects, though resembling crustaceans in many respects, are usually capable of more complex acts and also demand, if for no other reason than their number and that of their investigators, special treatment. The reader should therefore be aware that certain findings in one group of animals are not necessarily transferable to others.

REFERENCES

NICHOLLS, J. G., and D. A. BAYLOR, 1968. Specific modalities and receptive fields of sensory neurons in CNS of the leech. *J. Neurophysiol.* 31:740–756.

YOUNG, J. Z., 1971. *The Anatomy of the Nervous System of* Octopus vulgaris. London: Oxford University Press.

30 Comparisons between Vertebrates and Invertebrates in Nervous Organization

THEODORE HOLMES BULLOCK

ABSTRACT Some differences between vertebrate and higher invertebrate nervous systems are itemized. These concern myelin, dendrites, somata and concentrations of them, and neuropile and electrical activity. The control of muscle and several other physiological and anatomical items are alluded to.

The phenomenon of identifiable neurons is particularly discussed. It embraces both contrast and commonality between vertebrates and invertebrates. The claim is advanced that identifiable neurons are not peculiar to invertebrates or lower vertebrates. Three propositions are made: (1) In both vertebrates and invertebrates equivalence of neurons comes in various degrees, down to a few and even single, unique cells. (2) Among masses of neurons, formerly thought to be so nearly equivalent that large population statistics best characterize their actions, nonequivalent subsets and units will be discerned and more and more hierarchies will emerge. (3) There is no known prohibition that limits the integrative level to which the preceding propositions can operate. Some corollaries are stated.

WHY A SYMPOSIUM on invertebrate nervous systems in 1972? It is long since they needed to be sold or to have attention called to their advantageous preparations.

For my part, the reason for proposing and defending this topic is the conviction that besides important similarities there are significant contrasts between invertebrates and vertebrates in the organization of the substrates of behavior. How these contrasts are reflected in behavior, even to identify the contrasts satisfactorily let alone explain their consequences or adaptive significance, is still an exercise in groping, as it was in our treatise some years ago (Bullock and Horridge, 1965, pp. 10–24). But, on the eclectic principle that we cannot wait for one level of inquiry to be cleared up before proceeding at higher levels, it was my conviction that the special features of nervous organization in the higher protostomes—annelids, arthropods, and molluscs—justified a consideration of exemplary current work. Mutual exposure, I continue to hope, will build bridges across the unfortunate chasm often separating students of vertebrate and invertebrate nervous systems.

There are two hazards to this position, one on each side. Some colleagues, who are experts on vertebrates, expected the exercise to provide the elusive, ideal, "simple system." This is not altogether wrong, for an important spin-off, to be sure, is the advertisement of useful preparations. Other colleagues, on the other hand, including some of my fellow invertebrate zoologists, accuse me of infidelity for yielding to the siren song of vertebrates and even mammals! Such a one can no longer be trusted!

Rather than appealing to the record to make the case for following certain neural problems without regard to taxa or spines, this seems to be the place to plead guilty of the sin of comparing. I would like to lift up for emphasis just a few of the themes underlying our symposium and to place them in the perspective of general issues subsumed under the question: What can we say from vertebrate-invertebrate comparisons? Cohen (1970) has given a valuable essay on nearly the same theme in the last "Boulder volume."

I will not here catalog the extensive and profound *similarities* especially in signaling and integrative functions but will simply refer to Bullock and Horridge (1965). Time and again a feature discovered in one group and thought to be peculiar to it has then been found in the other—in both directions.

A. First, let us look at some *differences* between vertebrate and higher (more complex) invertebrate nervous organization.

1. Since some apparent exceptions have been resolved, it now seems correct to say that only vertebrates have true myelin—tightly and spirally wrapped, impeding current flow, forcing saltation and providing for conduction velocities five or ten times higher than the usual invertebrate maxima. (Shrimps achieve even higher velocity but

THEODORE HOLMES BULLOCK Department of Neurosciences, School of Medicine, and Neurobiology Unit, Scripps Institution of Oceanography, University of California, San Diego, La Jolla, California by a different means and without true myelin as defined. Amphioxus may have some myelin.)

2. With respect to afferent and integrative branches of neurons it seems likely—and, possibly, profoundly significant—that invertebrates essentially lack dendrites on the structural criteria for those processes in vertebrates for which the term was introduced. Invertebrate afferent processes are typically not made of cytoplasm so closely resembling that of the soma as is true in the vertebrates. Though some have short side branches, they are not readily equated with the spines of vertebrate dendrites. Invertebrate afferent processes do not arise from the soma but are borne on the axon or its collaterals. They are less profusely branched than many vertebrate dendrites and probably receive far fewer presynaptic contacts from far fewer types of impinging neurons, *as a rule* (i.e., overlapping frequency histograms but distinct modes).

I recommend a more rigorous usage of the term dendrite, returning to purely cytological defining characters as in the historical origin of the concept. This is a change from our former definition (Bullock and Horridge, 1965; see also Bodian, 1962), which mixed classical structural criteria and receptive and nonimpulse-conducting physiological criteria. Bodian and I now agree that advances in knowledge make the physiological criteria untenable for purposes of definition, although they are probably very common properties of many dendrites. True (cytological) dendrites can be both presynaptic and postsynaptic; receiving is commonplace in both somata and axons as well as dendrites; impulses can arise in or invade some good dendrites. The opening statement of the paragraph is based on this neoclassical definition that excludes receiving input as a defining criterion for dendrite. Invertebrate afferent processes or proximal or dendriform ramifications should be so termed, according to whether the context refers to functional or structural features, reserving dendrite for the case where one intends to imply that specified cytological criteria have been met. The first sentence of this paragraph is not meant to imply that we know enough to be at all confident of it. In fact it is striking how little we know of the cytology of proximal ramifications, or the localization of synaptic contacts, or the origin and limitation of impulses in invertebrates.

3. A significant difference in role of the perikaryon or cell body is closely related to the differences between the vertebrates and invertebrates in the cytology and the source of the afferent processes. In the invertebrates unipolar neurons are dominant and axosomatic synapses rare; the cell body is not in the path of excitation, is not needed for neural functions, and primarily serves to maintain the processes. Correspondingly, we see conspicuous histologic differences in central tissue, characteristic of these major divisions of the animal kingdom. Invertebrate ganglia have a central core of pure neuropil and a rind of cell bodies; vertebrates have gray matter in which the neuropil is usually broken up by cell bodies with axosomatic synapses. Here and there extensive neuropile, sparse in cell bodies (for example, molecular layer of cortex of cerebrum and cerebellum), is locally developed in vertebrates.

4. The ongoing electrical activity typical of higher centers in the two groups is possibly related to these general differences. Vertebrates have smooth, slow brain waves, as seen by macroelectrodes, almost without energy above 50 Hz, whether large mammal or tiny fish, whether with or without cortex, in highly ordered centers with geometrically regular arrays of cells and processes (cortex, hippocampus, etc.), and in centers not notable for such patterned structure (basal ganglia, hypothalamus, etc.). As seen by the same type of electrodes, invertebrates of many kinds in all three phyla sampled (annelids, arthropods, molluscs), with large or small brains, are typified by fast, spiky activity, very small slow waves, and plenty of energy above 100 Hz. (Cephalopods, for which we have only preliminary information, form a possible exception.) I suspect this is not due to size or number of cells but is a superficial manifestation of some important underlying difference inherent in items 2 and 3 above.

5. There are additional contrasts. The efferent control of muscle and integration in the periphery is a congeries of them. Degeneration and regeneration of motor axons is vastly different at least in some well-studied species, perhaps generally. Types of neurons, organelles and inclusions, types of glial cells, and vascular relations are generally different. The form and position of most sensory neurons is also, and the use of nonnervous sense cells in certain vertebrate receptors (acoustico-lateralis and taste) contrasts with the rule in invertebrates. Cephalization in invertebrates generally means movement of ganglia forward, whereas vertebrates add to existing rostral ganglia and shift functions forward—to oversimplify for the sake of brevity.

Note that the items of our list so far do not obviously predict, explain, or make sense in terms of general vertebrate-invertebrate differences in behavior or nervous achievement. The anatomical and physiological differences we know of to date do not themselves prove the existence of significant differences in integrative behavior, but they do strongly suggest that the mechanisms employed in integration are different in detail.

B. Let me now turn to a motif that played a prominent role in the chapters of this part and is often thought to be a feature of contrast between vertebrates and invertebrates, namely, the phenomenon of *identifiable neurons*. Identifiable neurons are unique cells that can be defined by distinguishing criteria, anatomical, chemical, and physiological and recognized in each individual of the species. Position of cell body is sometimes a good criterion, sometimes not. Processes and connections, cytoplasmic texture and pharmacologic type, synaptic responses, and spontaneous pattern are better criteria. Referring to the first of these, Pitman, Tweedle, and Cohen (1972) write "We are impressed by the precise reproduction of the branching pattern from one animal to the next for any given cell thus far examined." The number of identifiable neurons known is increasing every year and involves arthropods, molluscs, annelids, nematodes, and at least fish among the vertebrates.

The phenomenon of identifiable neurons embraces both contrast and commonality between vertebrates and invertebrates. In what degree or respect there is contrast is not yet known. The usual view today emphasizes the contrast, holding that vertebrates have large numbers of essentially equivalent and quite unreliable neurons operating probabilistically in masses (see Bullock, 1970). In this chapter I want to propose an important degree of *resemblance* between vertebrates and invertebrates, without denying at all that there may be important differences in respect to identifiable neurons.

Essentially, the claim I would like to advance is that (a) identifiable neurons are *not* peculiar to invertebrates or lower vertebrates but will also be found, with much greater difficulty of course, because of sheer numbers, in higher (more complex) forms and higher centers and that (b) other cells, though not individually identifiable, will be found to be essentially equivalent in larger and smaller groups down to very small numbers. For example, there are probably not many, if any, lateral geniculate or visual cortical cells with the same receptive field and the same size, threshold, contrast sensitivity, input-output function, time constants, and destination of axon. All of these would have to be the same for complete redundancy. A similar statement could be made for many other regions of the brain. Obviously, even if there were unique cells, this does not preclude overlapping properties; both can be graded from just barely to extensively.

Let me state the argument and its implications in the form of three propositions and their corollaries:

PROPOSITION 1: In both vertebrates and invertebrates equivalence of neurons comes in various degrees, from at least dozens of equivalent or virtually equivalent cells down to a few and even to zero equivalence (single, unique cells).

Corollaries:

(a) Nature does not require duplication of neurons.

(b) We may not assume as axiomatic that reserves against the contingency of injury or disease are an inevitable or ubiquitous good (in terms of survival value), stronger than opposing values, for example, for economy, adaptability or complexity.

(c) Large numbers of neurons do not necessarily mean high degrees of essential equivalence of neurons.

(d) Degrees of equivalence come in both dimensions: (1) gradation in numbers of fully equivalent cells and (2) gradation in equivalence (overlap of afferent fields and of efferent fields).

(e) Uniqueness of a unit may be due either to incomplete overlap of afferent field or of efferent field (or, of course, its transactional properties).

(f) All these statements apply to the highest and to the lowest nervous systems.

(g) The existence of potentially identifiable neurons is not antithetical to the highest vertebrate brains.

(h) Nothing is said or implied about the principles that govern or the facts of relative incidence of different degrees of equivalence in invertebrates vis à vis vertebrates. We cannot assume that even the direction of a preponderance, let alone the principles, are generally agreed to.

(i) The proposition predicts a one-way development of our knowledge, i.e., increasing numbers of instances of unique neurons and increasing discovery of differentiation among supposedly equivalent neurons even among vertebrates, and of course among invertebrates.

PROPOSITION 2: As masses of neurons are better understood and we sort them into nonequivalent subsets and units, not all of these will be hierarchically on a level but more and more hierarchies will emerge, with and without feedback. In other words, the prediction is that research on nucleus *X* will not only disprove the view that the population of cells is a mass of identical units with unspecified connections but will also reveal that some are higher than others in the same sense as Area 4 pyramidal cells are higher than ventral horn cells or Purkinje cells are higher than granule cells. The limitations of the concept of hierarchy are real, but the point here is that cells are likely to have nonparallel input and influence.

PROPOSITION 3: Working in from the periphery (*forward* from receptors, *backward* from effectors) to higher hierarchical levels, there is no known prohibition that limits the level to which the foregoing propositions can operate.

Corollaries:

(a) Nothing is said or implied about the principles or the facts of relative incidence of unique cells at higher and lower levels beyond the denial that such cells are a priori excluded.

(b) The proposition predicts a one-way development

of our knowledge, i.e., increasing numbers of instances of neurons with decreasing degrees of equivalence will be found *even at higher*, and of course at lower levels of all nervous systems.

These proposals represent severe extrapolations from the present state of knowledge. Nevertheless they are heuristic. The proposals not only suggest interesting lines of inquiry, but by their explicit statement, they also allow disproof or support of very general postulates by fragmentary evidence from special cases, as it comes in.

REFERENCES

Bodian, D., 1962. The generalized vertebrate neuron. *Science* 137:323–326.

Bullock, T. H., 1970. Reliability in neurons. *J. Gen. Physiol.* 55:565–584.

Bullock, T. H., and G. A. Horridge, 1965. *Structure and Function in the Nervous Systems of Invertebrates.* (2 vols.) San Francisco: W. H. Freeman & Company.

Cohen, M. J., 1970. A comparison of invertebrate and vertebrate central neurons. In *The Neurosciences: Second Study Program,* F. O. Schmitt, G. C. Quarton, T. Melnechuk, and G. Adelman, eds. New York: Rockefeller University Press, pp. 798–812.

Pitman, R. M., C. D. Tweedle, and M. J. Cohen, 1972. The form of nerve cells: Determination by cobalt impregnation. *Symposium on Staining Techniques in Neurobiology,* Iowa City, Iowa, 1972. New York: Springer-Verlag, (in press).

31 An Invertebrate System for the Cellular Analysis of Simple Behaviors and Their Modifications

ERIC R. KANDEL

ABSTRACT The abdominal ganglion of *Aplysia* controls several simple behaviors. One of these, the gill-withdrawal reflex, undergoes both short- and long-term behavioral modifications. Studies of the cellular bases of these behaviors and of their mechanisms of modification are reviewed.

Introduction

The study of the cellular mechanisms of behavior and its modification has recently received considerable impetus from two types of advances. One is the continuing improvement in techniques for analyzing the morphology, function, and biochemistry of individual nerve cells. The other is the utilization of the nervous systems of certain invertebrate animals (leeches, crayfish, lobsters, insects, and snails) that permit one to relate more directly the function of individual cells to behavior and to its modification. The central nervous systems of these invertebrates contain only 10^4 to 10^5 neurons, compared to the 10^{12} neurons of most vertebrates. Indeed some invertebrate ganglia contain only 1000 to 2000 neurons yet are capable of mediating several different behaviors so that the number of cells committed to a single behavior may be only 100 or less. Because of the small number of central neurons, the task of analyzing the functional architecture of behavior is significantly reduced. An additional advantage of invertebrates is that their nervous systems contain invariant cells that can be identified from preparation to preparation. The same cell can, therefore, be examined with the animal in different functional states.

As a result of these advantages, it is technically feasible in invertebrates to combine cellular neurophysiological and behavioral approaches and to attempt to clarify a number of interrelated neurophysiological and behavioral problems. For example, one can examine questions related to neuronal specialization. It is becoming evident that neurons may differ considerably in their physiological and biochemical properties. These differences are implied in the existence of uniquely identifiable cells. For what are these differences? Why are nervous systems not made up of identical units? By relating individual nerve cells to neural circuits controlling particular behaviors, one can examine how the distinctive properties of different types of neurons express themselves in mediating behavior. Using a combined approach, one can also examine behavioral questions. In particular one can analyze the relationships between behavioral modifications such as habituation and dishabituation, dishabituation and sensitization, and short-term and long-term memory. In the past, these processes have been compared only phenomenologically; with cellular techniques it may be possible to determine their mechanistic interrelationships.

By examining some of these questions I will here try to illustrate how studies of nerve cells and behavior can complement each other. I will first consider briefly some studies on neuronal specialization that have shown that different nerve cells and synapses have different plastic capabilities (for detailed reviews see Kandel and Spencer, 1968; von Baumgarten, 1970; Weight, this volume). Then I will consider recent experiments in a particular invertebrate, the marine mollusc *Aplysia*, which have delineated the neural circuits of two simple behaviors. One of the behaviors can be modified in several ways and provides an opportunity for examining the relationship of neuronal plasticity to behavioral modifications. Finally I will consider the mechanistic interrelationships between these behavioral modifications.

The plastic capabilities of neurons

Behavioral modifications require a prolonged, and sometimes a permanent change in neuronal function. How does this come about? As far as one can tell many connections between nerve cells are at least relatively specific.

ERIC R. KANDEL Department of Neurobiology and Behavior, The Public Health Research Institute of the City of New York; The Departments of Physiology and Psychiatry, New York University School of Medicine

They appear to be determined largely by genetic and developmental processes, and are present soon after birth (for alternative views on connection specificity see Sperry, 1965; Hubel and Wiesel, 1965; Gaze and Keating, 1972; and Blakemore, this volume). Furthermore, learning can occur quite rapidly often in a matter of minutes or seconds. These findings suggest that at least some forms of learning do not require the development of new nerve cells or the sprouting of new connections. It seems more likely that these forms of learning involve a change in the functional properties of previously existing cells or in the effectiveness of previously existing connections (Konorski, 1948; Hebb, 1949; Eccles, 1953; Kandel and Spencer, 1968). If this view is correct, we would expect that nerve cells or their synapses should be capable of changing their functional effectiveness and should show a certain amount of plasticity following repeated or patterned stimulation. Stated another way, if learning involves a change in the functional properties of neurons, then the very least we must demand is that some neurons show plastic capabilities.

This prediction has now been well supported: Work in a number of laboratories during the last three decades has shown that chemical (but not electrical) synapses can undergo a variety of plastic changes lasting minutes and even hours in response to repeated presynaptic stimulation (Larrabee and Bronk, 1947; del Castillo and Katz, 1954; Hughes, Evarts, and Marshall, 1956; Martin and Pilar, 1964; Kandel and Tauc, 1965b; Bruner and Tauc, 1966b; Spencer and April, 1970; Sherman and Atwood, 1971). Some synapses show facilitation, some show depression, some show facilitation at one frequency of stimulation and depression at other frequencies. Moreover, changes in synaptic plasticity can be homosynaptic or heterosynaptic. In homosynaptic plastic changes (posttetanic facilitation and depression; low-frequency facilitation and depression) the plastic change in functional effectiveness occurs in a given pathway as a result of a change in the frequency of activity in that pathway. In heterosynaptic plastic change (heterosynaptic facilitation and depression) the plastic change occurs in a pathway as a result of activity in another pathway.

The plastic capacities of neurons are not limited to their synaptic region. In certain instances the endogenous spike rhythms of pacemaker neurons can be modulated for relatively long periods of time and in other instances the thresholds of nonpacemaker neurons can change (Strumwasser, 1965; Frazier, Waziri and Kandel, 1965; Kandel, 1967; Stephens, 1972).

How can we relate these well-established instances of synaptic plasticity and other existing mechanisms of neuronal plasticity to behavior and behavioral modifications? To bridge this gap it is first necessary to develop suitable preparations in which behavior can be studied at the cellular level so that one can specify the neural circuit, or wiring diagram, that controls the behavior. This involves knowing which nerve cells control the different components of a behavioral sequence, and how these nerve cells interact with each other and with their respective sensory and motor neurons. Ultimately, it will also be important to know the transmitter biochemistry and synaptic morphology of all the cells that participate in the behavior. These stringent requirements cannot, at the moment, be satisfactorily met in the mammalian nervous system, although a good beginning is being made in several non-mammalian vertebrates (see for example Rovainen, 1967; Diamond, 1971; Martin and Wickelgren, 1971). However, these requirements are increasingly being met in certain arthropods, annelids, and molluscs (Kennedy, Selverston, and Remler, 1969; Nicholls and Purves, 1970; Kupfermann and Kandel, 1969).

To serve as a suitable preparation for relating behavioral modifications to cellular and synaptic processes, an invertebrate should be capable of generating interesting behaviors, comparable to those of vertebrates, and have a nervous system accessible to cellular analysis. For these reasons my colleagues Irving Kupfermann, Harold Pinsker, Vincent Castellucci, Thomas Carew, and I have worked on the role of one ganglionic complex, the abdominal ganglion, in controlling the behaviors of the marine mollusc *Aplysia*.

Aplysia is a large opisthobranch mollusc that generally lives only one year but grows to more than a foot in length and to several pounds in weight during its brief lifetime. This large marine snail has the four morphotypic features (Figure 1A4) that characterize the molluscan phylum: (1) a *head* carrying a mouth, tentacles, and eyes; (2) a *foot*; (3) a *mantle cavity*—a respiratory space containing the gill, and the discharge site for several excretory glands and for the renal and digestive systems; and (4) the *visceral* hump, which lies below the mantle cavity, and contains the heart, stomach, digestive gland and sexual apparatus. The mantle cavity and gill of *Aplysia* are covered by a protective layer, the *mantle shelf*, which contains a small, vestigial shell (Figure 1A1). The posterior margins of the mantle shelf are flared into a fleshy spout, the siphon, that serves as an exhalent funnel for sea water and debris circulating through the mantle cavity.

The *Aplysia* central nervous system contains about 15,000 to 20,000 neurons that are grouped into 9 major (and several minor) clusters called ganglia (Figure 1C1). Each ganglion contains only 1000 to 2000 neurons, yet individual ganglia are capable of generating specific behaviors. Eight of the nine major ganglia are symmetrical

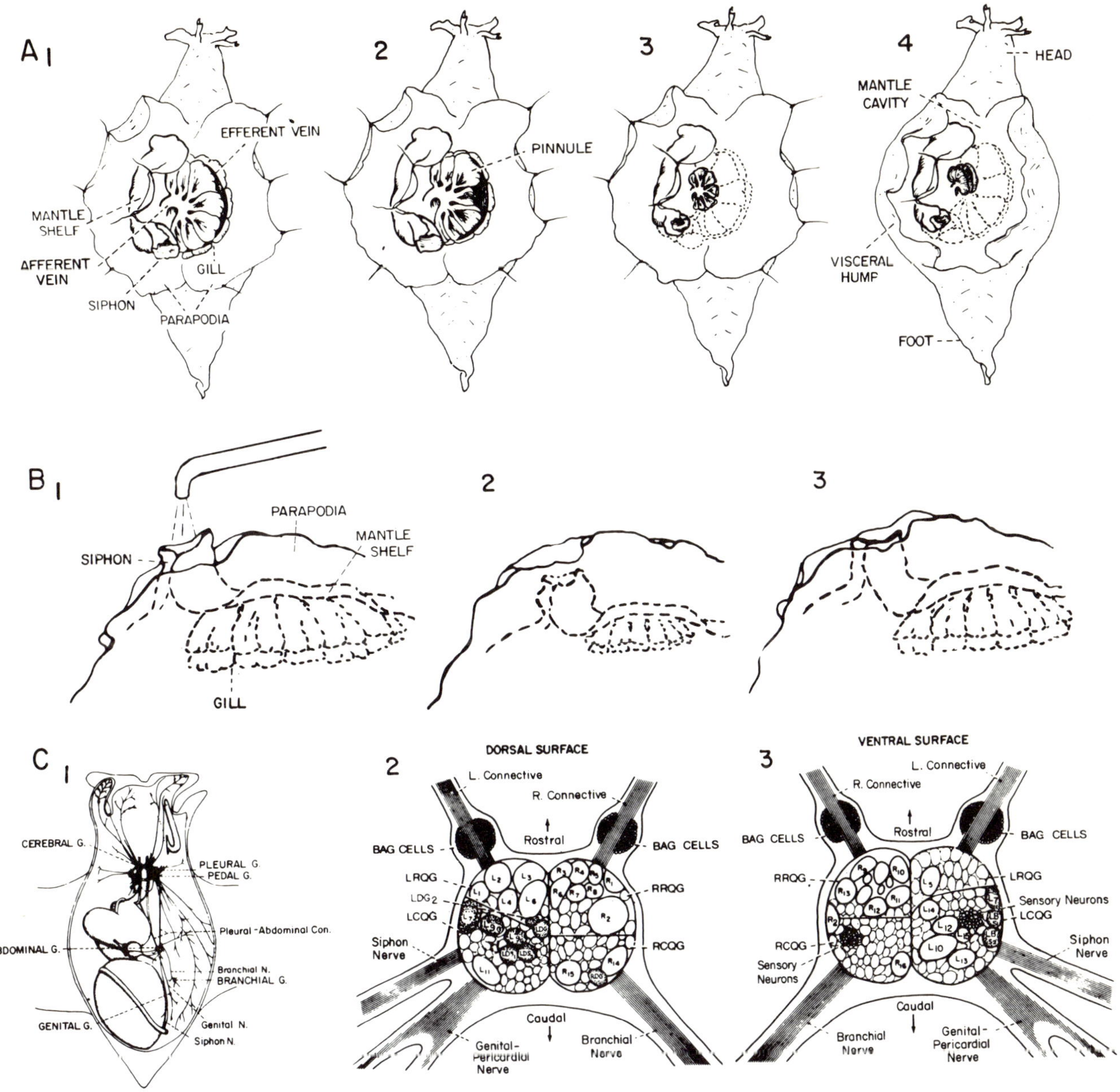

FIGURE 1 Different behaviors controlled by the abdominal ganglion of *Aplysia*. (A) Dorsal view of an intact *Aplysia* indicating the four features of the molluscan morphotype: Head, foot, mantle, and visceral hump (A4). To illustrate the three behaviors of the gill and siphon system, the parapodia and mantle shelf have been retracted so as to reveal the gill better. (A1) Position of organs in the unstimulated condition. (A2) The pinnule response to direct tactile stimulation of the gill. (A3) The defensive-withdrawal reflex to tactile stimulation of the siphon or mantle shelf. (A4) The centrally commanded gill, siphon and parapodial movements. (Modified from Kupfermann and Kandel, 1969; and Kupfermann, Pinsker, Castellucci, and Kandel, 1971). (B) Side view of an intact *Aplysia*, illustrating withdrawal of the siphon between the parapodia and the concomitant withdrawal of the gill into the mantle cavity during the defensive withdrawal reflex. The gill is seen through the parapodia. (C) The central nervous system of *Aplysia*. (C1) Four paired symmetrical (circumesophageal) ganglionic masses form a ring around the esophagus (the paired buccal, cerebral, pleural, and pedal ganglia); one ganglionic complex, the abdominal ganglion, lies below the esophagus. The circumesophageal ganglia innervate the head and foot. The abdominal ganglion innervates the mantle and its organs (gill, siphon, osphradium, purple and opaline glands) and the visceral hump (intestine, stomach, heart, sexual apparatus). The paired buccal ganglia are not indicated in the drawing; they lie on the ventral surface of the buccal mass, approximately in the position of the cerebral ganglia (from Eales, 1921). (C2) Dorsal and (C3) ventral views of the abdominal ganglion, illustrating identified cells (modified from Frazier, Waziri, and Coggeshall, 1967). The motor neurons for siphon and gill and the two sensory clusters have been stippled.

(paired cerebrals, buccals, pleurals and pedals) and form a *circumesophageal* ring of ganglia that control the organs of the head and foot. A single, ninth, unpaired *infraesophageal* or abdominal ganglion controls the organs of the mantle cavity and visceral hump. In addition to the central ganglia there also exists a peripheral nervous system that controls local responses (Bethe, 1903; Bullock and Horridge, 1965; Kandel and Spencer, 1968; Peretz, 1970; Kupfermann, Pinsker, Castellucci, and Kandel, 1971).

The cells of the *Aplysia* central nervous system are exceptionally large, particularly in the abdominal ganglion, where the smallest cells (50 to 70μ) are comparable to the larger cells in the mammalian brain and the largest cells reach almost 1 mm in diameter (Figures 1C2, 1C3). These giant cells of opisthobranch nervous systems are the largest known nerve cell bodies. Because of their size, they are easy to impale with microelectrodes, and one can readily record from, or stimulate, several cells simultaneously. They can also be individually dissected for biochemical studies (Giller and Schwartz, 1968, 1971a, 1971b; McCaman and Dewhurst, 1970; Wilson, 1970; Lasek and Dower, 1971). Some cells are so characteristic in their position, appearance, and electrophysiological, morphological and biochemical properties (Figures 1C1, 1C2) that they can be reliably identified from preparation to preparation (Arvanitaki and Tchou, 1942; Arvanitaki and Chalazonitis, 1958; Frazier et al., 1967). These advantages have made *Aplysia* useful for studying the biophysical properties of nerve cells (Tauc, 1962, 1966; Strumwasser, 1967, this volume), the pharmacology and biochemistry of synaptic transmission (Tauc, 1967; Tauc and Gerschenfeld, 1961; Kandel, 1968; Kehoe, 1972), and the plastic properties of neurons and synapses (Kandel and Tauc, 1965a; Bruner and Tauc, 1966b; Strumwasser, 1967; Bruner and Kehoe, 1970). Recently it has also proved possible to map the interconnections between neurons in *Aplysia* ganglia on a cell-to-cell basis (Kandel, Frazier, Waziri, and Coggeshall, 1967; Kehoe, 1969; Gardner, 1971; Gardner and Kandel, 1972). This permits one to examine how cells are connected to each other and to the sensory and motor periphery, and to evaluate, at times quantitatively, what a given cell contributes to a particular behavior. I will consider below one well-studied example of a cellular analysis of behavior.

The gill and siphon of Aplysia: *Multiple controls of a single effector system*

The simple behaviors of vertebrates and invertebrates can be divided into two classes: (1) reflexive behavior; and (2) centrally initiated (or commanded) behavior (see Thorpe, 1963; Hinde, 1970). A reflex behavior is elicited by a specific sensory stimulus, and its response amplitude is a function of the intensity of the sensory stimulus. A centrally commanded behavior can occur spontaneously or can be triggered by a sensory stimulus. When triggered, the response amplitude is independent of stimulus strength. Because the amplitude and sequence of these responses are preprogrammed, centrally commanded behaviors are often called "fixed action patterns" (Tinbergen, 1951).

Some effector systems can be controlled both reflexly and by central commands. The siphon and gill system of *Aplysia* is of this type and provides a useful preparation for examining the interrelationships of reflexive and centrally commanded behaviors. This system also turns out to be useful for comparing behaviors mediated by the central nervous system and peripherally mediated local responses, characteristic of molluscs.

As described earlier, the gill of *Aplysia* is housed in the mantle cavity that is covered by a fold of skin, the mantle shelf (Figure 1A1). Posteriorly the mantle shelf forms a fleshy spout, the siphon, that normally protrudes from the mantle cavity between the parapodia, the wing-like extensions of the foot (Figures 1A1, 1B1). The gill is a large external respiratory organ composed of about 16 individual pinnules supplied by an afferent and an efferent vein. When the siphon or the mantle shelf is touched, both the siphon and the gill withdraw reflexly into the mantle cavity (Figures 1A3, 1B2). As the gill withdraws its volume is reduced, its halves tend to close and the pinnules separate slightly (Figure 1A3). This response has the features of a simple defensive withdrawal reflex; it has a short latency and its amplitude is a function of the intensity of the tactile stimulus. This reflex permits the animal to respond to a potentially threatening stimulus by withdrawing gill and siphon into the mantle cavity where they are protected by the mantle shelf and the parapodia. The contraction of the gill and siphon occur concomitantly so that observing one component of the system provides an index of the activity of the other component. This is convenient because gill movement can only be measured in restrained animals in which the parapodia and mantle shelf are retracted to expose the gill (Figure 2B). Siphon movements can be measured, however, in the completely unrestrained animal (Figure 1B).

In response to a central command from the abdominal ganglion, a superficially similar but actually quite different behavioral response occurs (Figure 1A4). It consists of a contraction with reduction of gill volume, accompanied by rostral rotation of the gill, bunching together of the pinnules and separation of the two gill halves (flaring) exposing the efferent vein. The parapodia

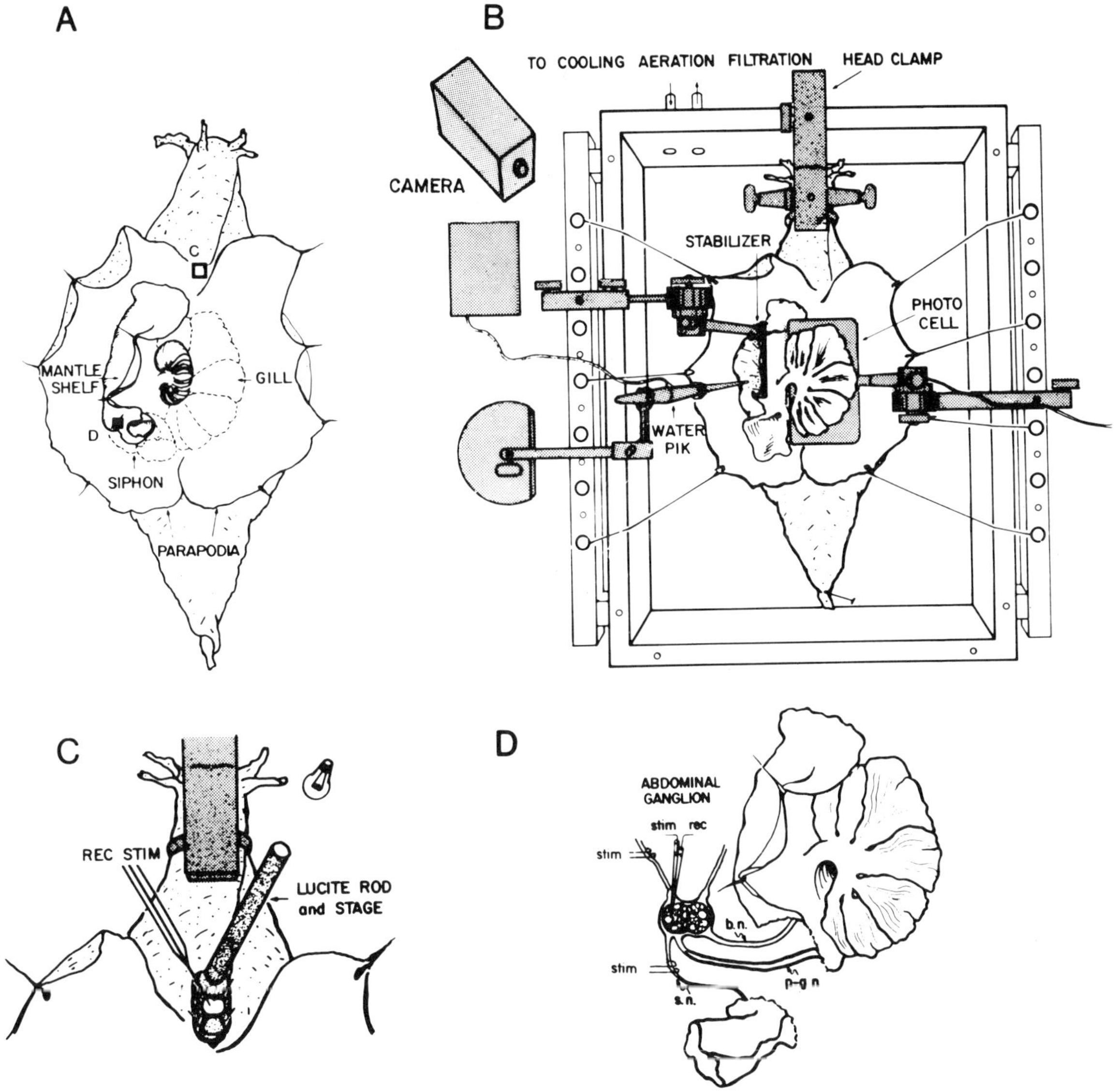

FIGURE 2 Different preparations used to study gill and siphon withdrawal reflexes. (A) Dorsal view of the intact animal with parapodia and mantle shelf retracted. (B) Experimental set-up for behavioral studies of gill withdrawal in the intact animal. *Aplysia* immobilized in a small aquarium containing cooled, filtered and aerated circulating sea water. The edge of the mantle shelf is pinned to a substage and a constant and quantifiable tactile stimulus is delivered by brief jets of sea water from a commercially available Water Pik. The behavioral responses were monitored with a photocell placed under the gill or by means of 16 mm movies (modified from Pinsker et al., 1970). (C) Preparation for simultaneous study of cellular and behavioral responses. Intact animal immobilized as in (B). A small slit is made at the most posterior end of the spermatic groove (see C in A), and the abdominal ganglion with its peripheral nerves and connectives intact is externalized and pinned to a lucite stage. Identified motor cells impaled with double-barrelled microelectrodes for intracellular stimulation and recording. Gill movements recorded with photocell and camera (from Kupfermann et al., 1970). (D) Test system of gill-withdrawal reflex in isolated abdominal ganglion. In some cases, the abdominal ganglion remained connected to the gill via the branchial (b.n.) and pericardial-genital (p-g.n.) nerves and to the siphon via the siphon nerve (s.n.). Intracellular recordings are obtained from motor neurons (usually L7); tactile stimuli are applied to the siphon skin or electrical stimuli to the siphon nerve or connective. (Modified from Castellucci et al., 1970.)

also often contract, forcing sea water through the mantle cavity. These spontaneous contractions sometimes recur at intervals of several minutes and serve to pump sea water through the mantle cavity thereby aerating the gill and cleansing the cavity.

In addition to these two behavioral sequences, individual pinnules of the gill contract when a tactile stimulus is applied to them directly (Figure 1A2). The receptive field of the pinnule response is centered on the pinnule itself. The strongest contraction occurs immediately under the site of stimulation (Peretz, 1970; Kupfermann, Pinsker, Castellucci, and Kandel, 1971).

To relate these behaviors to cellular neuronal mechanisms four different preparations have been used. The *first* is a completely intact unrestrained animal in which siphon responses to natural stimuli can be measured (Figures 1B, 2A). The *second* preparation is an intact animal restrained in a small aquarium, containing cooled circulating sea water, in which gill responses to natural stimuli can be measured by means of a photocell. For a more detailed and qualitative analysis, motion pictures can be taken of gill movements (Figure 2B). Quantifiable and constant tactile stimuli are provided by jets of sea water from a Water Pik. The *third* preparation is an intact animal prepared as above, but with a slit in its neck (Figure 2C) through which the abdominal ganglion is externalized and gill responses and intracellular responses from single nerve cells are recorded or photographed simultaneously. The *fourth* preparation consists of the isolated abdominal ganglion with or without the siphon skin and gill and can be used as a test system of the behavior for more detailed cellular studies (Figure 2D).

GILL MOTOR NEURONS *The movements produced by different motor neurons* The motor components of the reflex response and of the centrally commanded movement (Figure 2C) were investigated in the intact preparation with a slit in the animal's neck (Kupfermann and Kandel, 1968, 1969; Kupfermann, Carew, and Kandel, 1973). One or more nerve cells were impaled with microelectrodes and stimulated with intracellular current pulses while the movements of the different external organs of the mantle cavity were monitored with a photocell and, in some cases, with a 16mm movie camera. Six cells were found—five in the left caudal quarter-ganglion (L7, LD_{G1}, LD_{G2}, $L9_{G1}$, and $L9_{G2}$) and one in the right caudal quarter-ganglion (RD_G)—that produced movements of the gill (Figures 1C2, 1C3, 3A; see also Peretz, 1969). Stimulation of three cells (L7, LD_{G1}, and LD_{G2}) produced particularly large and brisk gill movements. The other three cells ($L9_{G1}$, $L9_{G2}$, and RD_G) produced smaller contractions.

Stimulation of L7 typically elicits a gill contraction that results in a great reduction in volume and concomitant closure of the two gill halves with separation of the pinnules at their base (Figure 1A3). Cells $L9_{G1}$ and $L9_{G2}$ produce similar but weaker movements. Like L7, stimulation of LD_{G1} also causes a large contraction with a great reduction of volume, but it also causes rostral rotation of the gill and bunching together of the pinnules. Stimulation of LD_{G2} produces flaring of the two gill halves (Figure 1A4); RD_G produces similar but weaker movements. Thus the two different gill behaviors are based on the characteristic movements produced by the three major motor cells L7, LD_{G1}, and LD_{G2}. The reduction in gill volume and separation of the pinnules with no flaring or even antiflaring of the gill halves, characteristic of the defensive reflex, is based upon the combined actions of all three cells with the L7 actions slightly predominant. The reduction in gill volume with rostral rotation, bunching of the pinnules, and flaring of the two gill halves characteristic of the central command is based upon the unopposed actions of LD_{G1} and LD_{G2} with the actions of LD_{G2} usually predominant.

Four neurons in the left caudal quarter-ganglion (LB_{S1}, LB_{S2}, LD_{S1}, and LD_{S2}) were found to be specific for siphon contraction. In addition, the gill motor neuron L7 also causes contraction of the siphon as well as of the mantle shelf. The motor component of the total defensive withdrawal reflex thus consists of at least ten cells, organized in a hierarchical pattern. Five of the ten motor cells produce movements limited to the gill (LD_{G1}, LD_{G2}, RD_G, $L9_{G1}$, and $L9_{G2}$). Four cells produce movements largely limited to the siphon (LB_{S1}, LB_{S2}, LD_{S1}, and LD_{S2}) and one cell (L7) produces movements of the gill, siphon, and mantle shelf. Thus, the motor components of this reflex consist of individual elements with both a restricted and an overlapping distribution.

Neuromuscular connections of gill motor neurons All six motor cells to the gill send their axons out of the ganglion via peripheral nerves to innervate the gill. To determine whether the major motor neurons produced their effect directly on gill muscle or via peripheral interneurons in the gill itself, Carew, Pinsker, Rubinson, Schwartz, and Kandel (1973) studied the neuromuscular connections of the major motor cells, L7, LD_{G1}, and LD_{G2}. They impaled motor neurons in the ganglion, and individual muscle fibers in the walls of the efferent or afferent blood vessel of the gill, and found that action potentials in each of the motor neurons produced excitatory junction potentials (EJPs) in the muscle fibers (Figures 3B1, 3B2). These EJPs followed the motor neuron spikes one for one up to relatively high frequencies (15/sec). The latencies of the EJPs were constant even in high Ca^{++} solutions that would raise the threshold of interneurons.

These results indicated that these major motor neurons innervate gill muscle directly. The junctions are chemical and are reversibly blocked by sea water solutions containing high Mg^{++}. The neuromuscular connections of the three minor motor neurons have not yet been examined.

The chemical transmitters produced by LD_{G1} and L7 As a beginning in the study of the transmitter biochemistry of the motor cells for gill movement, Carew, Schwartz, and Kandel (1972) examined the biochemical and pharmacological properties of LD_{G1} and L7. They found that the gill contraction caused by LD_{G1} is reversibly inhibited by hexamethonium, which blocks the excitatory actions of acetylcholine (ACh) in *Aplysia* (Tauc and Gerschenfeld, 1961). By contrast hexamethonium did not affect the contractions produced by L7. These results suggested that LD_{G1} is cholinergic and that L7 is not. Moreover, when the cells were dissected from the ganglion and assayed for the presence of choline acetyl-transferase, the enzyme required for the synthesis of ACh, cell LD_{G1} was found to contain the transferase whereas L7 did not. Next, radioactive choline was injected into the cell body of L7 or LD_{G1} to determine the amount of radioactive choline that each cell converted to ACh. In L7 the ^{3}H-choline was converted to substances other than ACh, predominantly phosphoryl choline, but in LD_{G1} 85% of the choline was converted to acetylcholine. Taken together, the pharmacological and biochemical data support the idea that LD_{G1} is cholinergic and L7 is not.

Some muscle fibers were found to receive EJPs from each of these two cells (Figure 3B3). This finding suggests that two excitatory motor neurons, using different chemical transmitters, can make direct connections with the same muscle fiber. However, the possibility that L7 and LD_{G1} innervate different fibers, which are electrically coupled, is not ruled out.

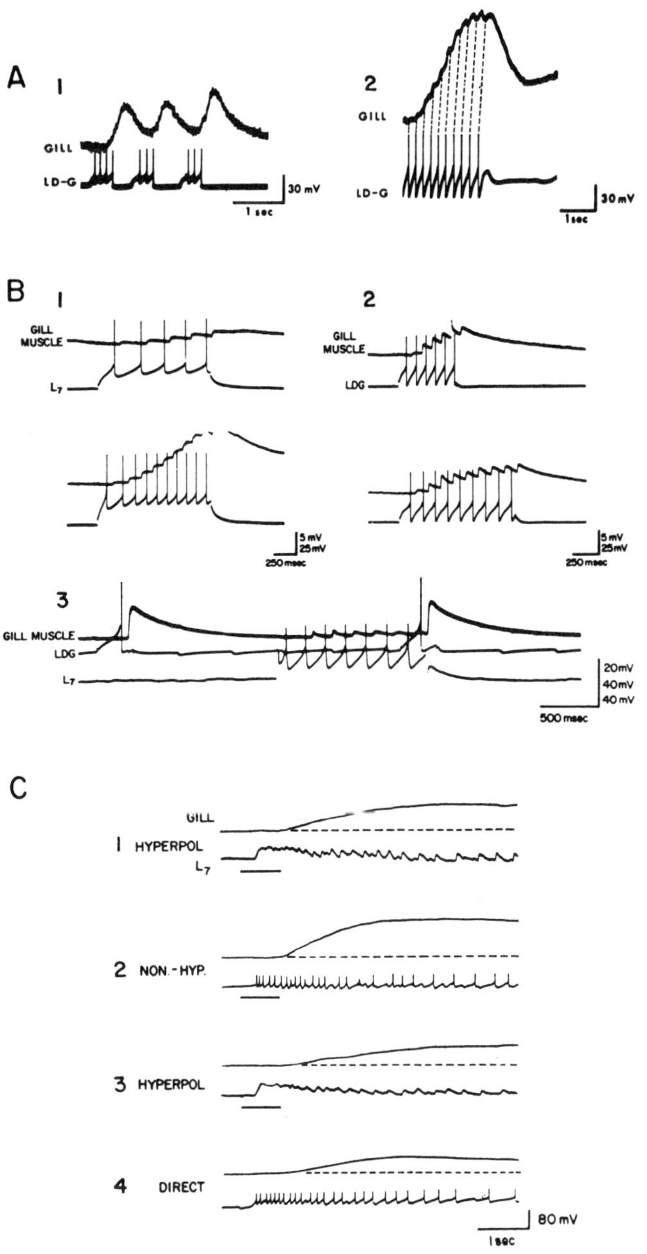

FIGURE 3 Responses of gill and individual gill muscle fibers to stimulation of individual motor cells and sensory input. (A) Response of the gill. Upper traces represent the output of a photocell placed under the gill, lower traces intracellular recordings from a motor neuron causing gill contraction. (A1) Smooth contraction produced by small number of spikes in cell LD_{G1}. (A2) Individual twitches produced by LD_{G1} after it was first stimulated at high frequency to potentiate its effects. (From Kupfermann and Kandel, 1969.) (B) Intracellular recordings of excitatory junction potentials (EJPs) in gill muscle fibers (top trace) due to intracellular stimulation of L7 or LD_{G1} (bottom traces). (B_1) Spikes in L7 were elicited by depolarizing pulses of different intensities. The EJPs in the gill followed L7 spikes one for one with a fixed latency at both low frequencies (5/sec) and higher frequencies (10/sec). At the higher frequency the EJPs potentiate. (B2) Response of gill muscle fiber to intracellular stimulation of LD_{G1}. (B3) Intracellular recording from LD_{G1}, L7, and a single muscle fiber showing two types of EJPs, one from LD_{G1} and the other from L7. (From Carew, Pinsker, Schwartz, Rubinson and Kandel, 1973.) (C) The sensory input to the gill motor neuron. The gill-withdrawal reflex was elicited every 5 min by a jet of sea water (indicated by solid line, under L7 record) applied to the siphon. Hyperpolarization of L7 on alternate trials (C1 and C3) unmasked the large excitatory synaptic input that normally underlies the repetitive discharge (C2). Comparisons of hyperpolarized to nonhyperpolarized trials showed that the gill contraction was reduced by about 40%. This reduction was approximately equal to the size of the gill contraction produced by L7 when it was fired intracellularly by a long depolarizing pulse (C4) that caused L7 to fire in a pattern comparable to that produced by the normal excitatory input. (From Kupfermann, Pinsker, Castellucci, and Kandel, 1971.)

The Sensory Input to Gill Motor Neurons Causing Defensive Withdrawal Reflex To study the sensory input to motor neurons Kupfermann and Kandel (1969) and Kupfermann, Pinsker, Castellucci, and Kandel (1971) stimulated the body surface of the animal with tactile stimuli while recording from gill motor neurons, one at a time. These tactile stimuli produced excitatory postsynaptic potentials (EPSPs) in each of the motor neurons that caused the cell to fire repetitively (Figure 3C). The receptive fields of the motor neurons were identical with that for the gill-withdrawal reflex.

To examine the EPSPs the motor neuron was hyperpolarized to prevent spike generation. In this way, the gill contraction to a constant siphon stimulus could be measured under two conditions: (1) with the motor neuron at its resting potential and firing normally (Figure 3C2), and (2) with the motor neuron selectively removed from the reflex pathway by hyperpolarizing it to prevent spike generation (Figures 3C1, 3C3). By seeing how much the gill contraction was reduced by the temporary removal of one cell from the reflex pathway, it was possible to determine the relative contributions of the individual motor neurons to the total gill-withdrawal reflex. This could be checked by showing that when the motor neuron was fired by intracellular depolarization, in a manner that simulated its synaptic activation during the reflex (Figure 3C), the gill movement produced was comparable to that component of the total reflex response that was removed when the motor neuron was hyperpolarized. By this means, the average contribution of L7 was estimated to be 35 to 40%, and that of LD_{G1} about 30 to 35%. The contractions produced by LD_{G1} and L7 were additive. Thus, these two cells account for a major portion of the total reflex. Each of the other motor neurons (LD_{G2}, RD_G, $L9_{G1}$, and $L9_{G2}$) contributes less to the reflex contractions, but their quantitative contributions have not yet been determined.

The reflexly produced EPSPs unmasked in these motor neurons by hyperpolarization (Figures 3C1, 3C3) are due to the activity of both monosynaptic and polysynaptic pathways. The monosynaptic contribution from the siphon and mantle shelf is mediated by two distinctive clusters of sensory neurons. One of these is located in the left caudal quarter-ganglion near the motor neurons (Figure 1B2) and conveys tactile information from the siphon skin via the siphon nerve. The other is located in the right caudal quarter-ganglion and conveys tactile input from the mantle shelf via the branchial nerve (Castellucci, Pinsker, Kupfermann, and Kandel, 1970; Byrne, Castellucci, and Kandel, 1973). Only the cluster containing the siphon sensory cells has been studied in detail. Each of these sensory neurons has about the same threshold to mechanical stimulation and a rather discrete receptive field. At least some of the fields are invariant. The receptive fields fall into three size classes: Some fields are small, covering about 20% of the siphon skin; some are medium sized, covering about 40% of the siphon skin; and two are large, covering 80% of the siphon. Thus, like the motor neurons, the sensory neurons are arranged in a field size hierarchy.

The sensory neurons from the siphon skin connect to the motor neurons directly (Figure 4A). In addition, they connect to three types of interneurons (Figure 4B). Two of these are excitatory (Figure 4B1), and produce EPSPs in motor neuron L7. One interneuron, cell L16, is inhibitory (Figure 4B2). It inhibits the sensory neurons as well as other interneurons (Castellucci and Kandel, in preparation).

Synaptic Input to Gill Motor Neurons During Centrally Commanded Gill Movements During defensive withdrawal all the gill motor cells fire synchronously (Figure 4C1) but during the centrally commanded movement, they fire in a specific sequence (Figure 4C2). The central command manifests itself at the level of the motor neurons as a characteristic PSP burst (Kupfermann and Kandel, 1968, 1969; Peretz, 1969). This is attributed to the activity of several closely coupled interneurons, one of which is Interneuron II (Kandel et al., 1967). The PSP burst does not require sensory feedback from the gill for its generation and can occur in the completely isolated abdominal ganglion (Waziri and Kandel, 1969). In LD_{G1}, LD_{G2}, and RD_G, the PSP burst consists of EPSPs that produce excitation. In LD_{G1}, the EPSP burst is preceded by a brief period of inhibition (Figure 4C2). In the three other motor cells (L7, $L9_{G1}$, $L9_{G2}$), the PSP burst consists of IPSPs that produce inhibition followed by rebound. The rebound excitation adds to the last stages of the contraction. Synaptic inhibition therefore provides a means for sequencing the firing of the motor neurons so that the discharge of LD_{G2} and RD_G precedes that of LD_{G1}, which in turn precedes that of L7, $L9_{G1}$, and $L9_{G2}$. As a consequence, a pumping action can be produced that seems to circulate blood through the gill while the concomitant parapodial contractions move fresh water through the mantle cavity.

The siphon motor neurons are also excited in synchrony by the defensive reflex and differentially excited (LD_{S1} and LD_{S2}) and inhibited (L7, LB_{S1}, and LB_{S2}) during the central command.

Neural Circuits of the Defensive-Withdrawal Reflex and the Centrally Commanded Movements The above results allow a wiring diagram for both reflex and centrally commanded responses to be drawn

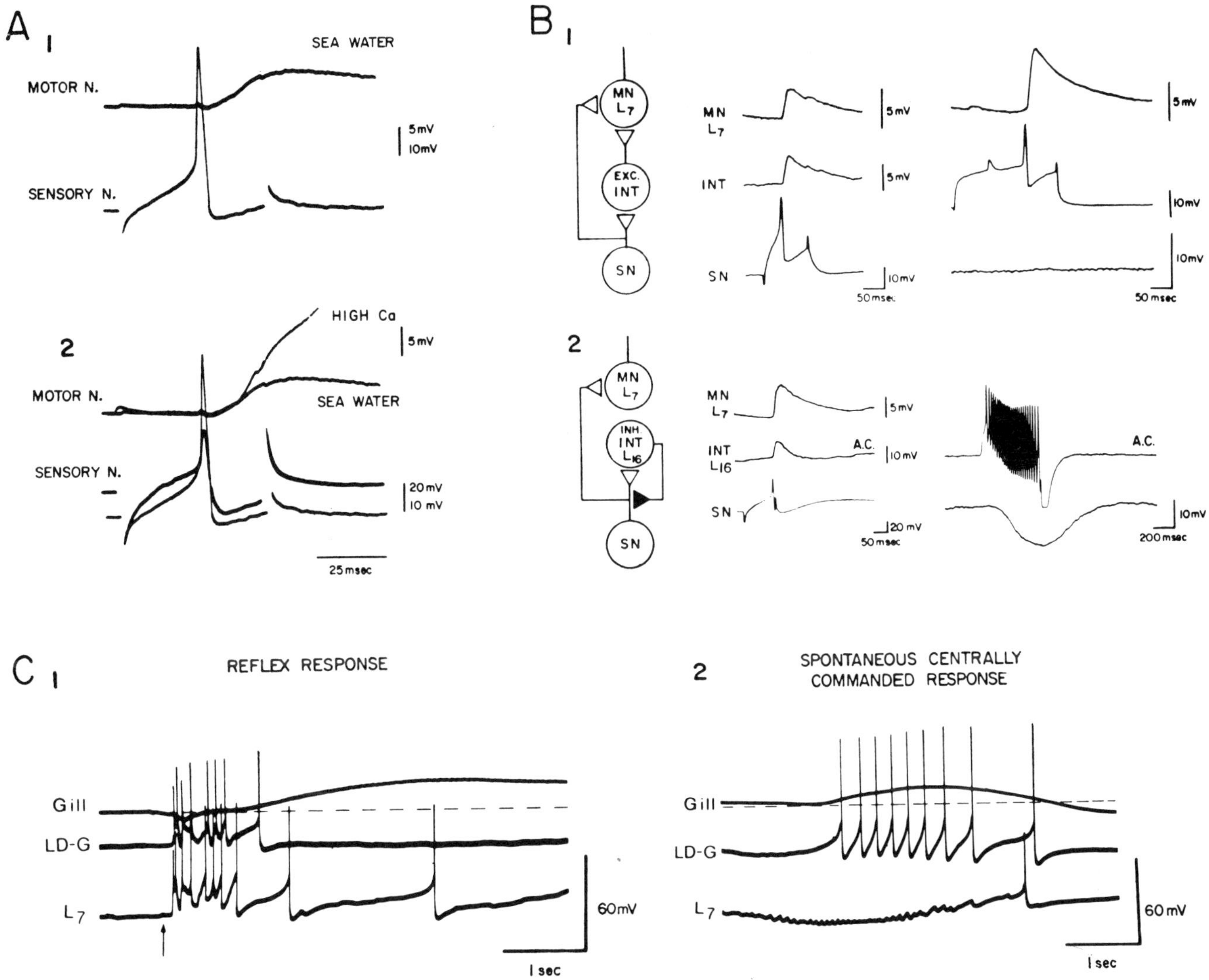

FIGURE 4 The synaptic input for the (A–C1) gill-withdrawal reflex and for the (C2) centrally commanded gill movements. (A) The EPSP in gill motor neuron L7 produced by intracellular stimulation of a sensory neuron. (A1) Fast sweep recording to illustrate the short latency of the EPSP. (A2) Superimposed traces of EPSP elicited in artificial sea water with normal Ca^{++} content (9.1 mM) and in a solution of high Ca^{++} content (91 mM). Because of the increased threshold in high Ca^{++}, the intracellular stimulation had to be increased considerably, resulting in a large current artifact that could not be completely balanced with the Wheatstone bridge; the gain was therefore reduced (see calibration). The latency of the EPSP remained the same. (From Carew, Castellucci, and Kandel, 1971.) (B) Central connections of sensory neurons (SN) with interneurons. (B1) Intracellular stimulation of sensory neuron produces an EPSP in an excitatory interneuron (middle). An action potential in the excitatory interneuron, in turn, causes an excitatory potential in the motor neuron L7 (right). These connections are summarized in the drawing on the left. (B2) Intracellular stimulation of a sensory neuron produces an EPSP in inhibitory interneuron L16 (middle column). Repetitive discharge of the interneuron inhibits this and other sensory neurons as shown by the hyperpolarization (right). These connections are summarized in the drawing on the left. (From Castellucci and Kandel, in preparation.) (C) Comparison of synaptic input to L7 and LD_{G1} during gill-withdrawal reflex (C1) and centrally commanded contraction (C2). (From Kupfermann and Kandel, 1969.)

(Figures 5A, 5B1). The mechanoreceptor sensory neurons involved in the defensive withdrawal reflex make excitatory connections with both gill and siphon motor neurons directly and indirectly via excitatory interneurons (Figure 5B1). In addition, they connect with an inhibitory interneuron which feeds back on the sensory neurons and forward to the excitatory interneurons. In the spontaneous movements (Figure 5A) the central command elements excite some gill and siphon motor neurons and inhibit others. The central command interneurons can fire spontaneously but also receive either a direct or indirect excitatory input from the siphon and the mantle shelf. Thus, as a result of multiple synaptic inputs, the different members of the same population of motor cells can be switched between either a simple reflex or a centrally commanded behavior.

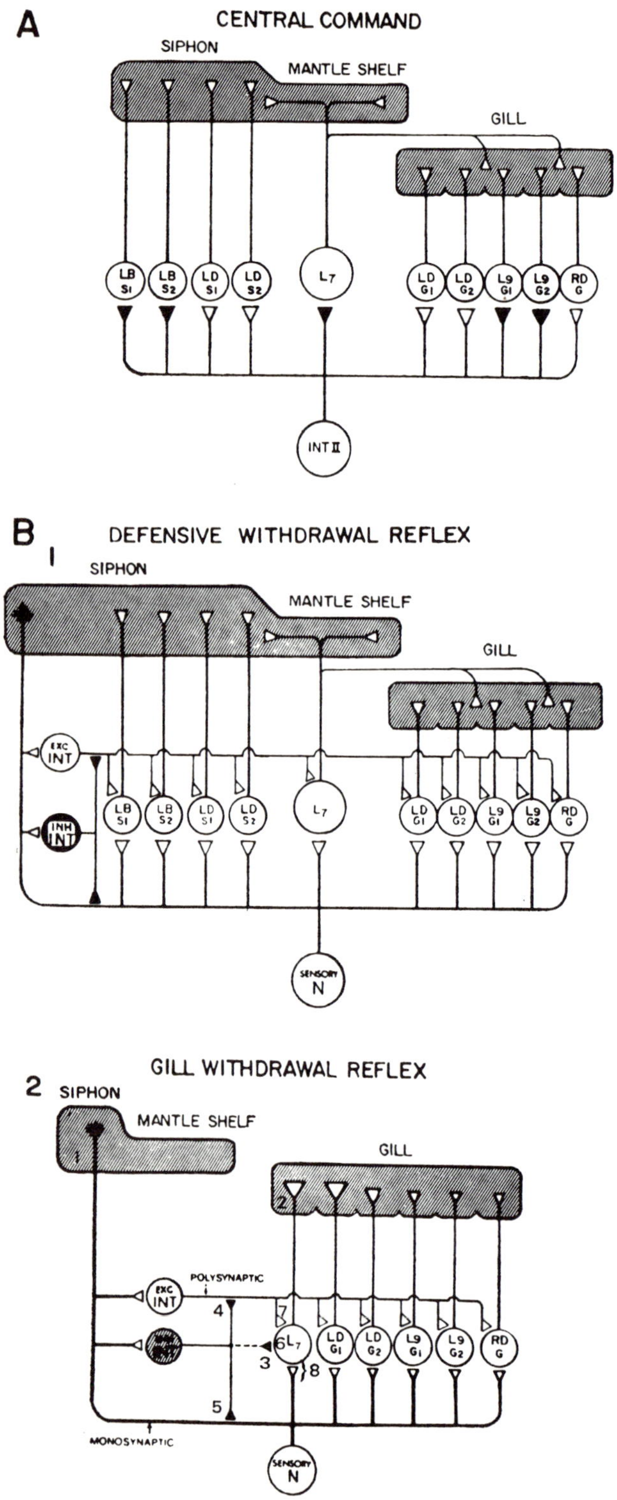

Two main findings are illustrated by these circuit diagrams. (1) The various motor neurons of the mantle organs are independent, parallel elements that are not interconnected with each other. (2) Both motor neurons and sensory neurons are arranged in a hierarchical manner. Some sensory neurons receive from small areas of siphon skin, some from medium sized areas, and one cell receives from the whole siphon. Similarly, some motor neurons move only the gill, some move only the siphon, and one moves the siphon together with the gill and mantle shelf. As a result of these two factors, reflex actions or central commands can play on different combinations of a common motor pool to generate different behavioral combinations and different temporal sequences of the same combination. This permits an effector organ, or a whole effector system, to be controlled in a number of different ways. In addition, the whole mantle system (gill, siphon, and mantle shelf) can also be controlled in different combinations with other effector systems, such as heart and kidney (Mayeri, Kupfermann, Koester, and Kandel, 1971).

Whereas Figure 5B1 illustrates the total defensive withdrawal reflex, Figure 5B2 illustrates the neural circuit of the gill component on which is based most of the work considered below.

THE RELATIONSHIP OF THE PINNULE RESPONSE TO THE GILL-WITHDRAWAL REFLEX Since both pinnule response and gill-withdrawal reflex involve movements of the gill, it became of interest to compare them to see whether they involve similar or different processes (Peretz, 1970). The gill-withdrawal reflex is elicited by stimulating not the gill itself but a remote receptive field

FIGURE 5 Neural system controlling centrally commanded gill movements and defensive withdrawal reflex. Dark triangles indicate inhibition; light triangles, excitation. (A) Centrally commanded gill movements. Interneuron II probably represents several closely coupled interneurons which excite some gill and siphon motor neurons (RD_G, LD_{G1}, LD_{G2}, LD_{S1}, LD_{S2}) and inhibit others ($L9_{G1}$, $L9_{G2}$, L7, LB_{S1}, LB_{S2}). (B) Defensive withdrawal reflex. (B1) The total reflex, illustrating both siphon and gill components. (B2) The gill-withdrawal component of the reflex. The sensory input from the siphon is mediated directly and via interneurons. (Exc. Int. and Sensory N represent classes of cells.) Motor neurons and inhibitory interneurons are identified cells. Small numbers indicate possible sites of plasticity. The large triangles represent the output of major motor cells that contribute importantly to the gill withdrawal, small triangles that of cells producing weaker effects. In this, and subsequent figures, synapses are schematically indicated as being on the cell body. Actually they are on the initial segment of the axon and its branches. (Modified from Kupfermann and Kandel, 1969; Kupfermann, Carew, and Kandel, 1973.)

consisting of the siphon and mantle shelf (Figures 1A3, 1B1). This reflex is centrally mediated. When individual central motor neurons are hyperpolarized and prevented from spiking so that their contributions to the reflex are eliminated, the total reflex is significantly reduced (Figure 3C1). When chemical synaptic transmission in the abdominal ganglion is reversibly blocked by bathing it in a solution of isotonic magnesium chloride, the reflex response to moderate tactile stimuli is fully but reversibly blocked (Kupfermann et al., 1971). Surgical removal of the ganglion also eliminates the gill-withdrawal reflex. However, when the siphon is surgically isolated from the rest of the animal and left attached to the abdominal ganglion by only the siphon nerve (Figure 2D), so that the central pathways are preserved while parallel peripheral pathways via the skin are totally eliminated, tactile stimulation of the siphon still produces a brisk gill-withdrawal reflex.

The pinnule response differs from the gill-withdrawal reflex in several ways. First, the most effective site for eliciting the pinnule response is not a remote site but the gill pinnule itself (Figure 1A2). Second, although the pinnule response can be elicited in the intact animal, it can also be elicited when all central ganglia are removed. This indicates that central pathways are not necessary for the pinnule response. The response is mediated by peripheral pathways either by the neurons in the gill, by collaterals of central neurons, or by direct stimulation of the muscle itself (Peretz, 1970; Kupfermann, Pinsker, Castellucci, and Kandel, 1971).

Neural plasticity and behavioral modifications of the gill-withdrawal reflex: Habituation and dishabituation

Since gill (and siphon) movements occur spontaneously as well as reflexly, they are, in principle, amenable to both operant and classical conditioning training procedures. To begin the study of behavioral modifications of this system, Pinsker, Kupfermann, Castellucci, and Kandel (1970) and Carew, Pinsker, and Kandel (1972) focused on the reflex response and utilized an even simpler behavioral paradigm, habituation and dishabituation.

Habituation, sometimes considered the most elementary form of learning, is a decrease in a behavioral response that occurs when an initially novel stimulus is presented repeatedly (Figure 6A). When a novel stimulus, such as a sudden noise, is presented for the first time, attention is immediately drawn to it and one's heart rate and respiratory rate may increase. However, if the same noise is repeated, one's attention, as well as one's bodily responses, gradually diminish. As a result of habituation, one can become accustomed to initially distracting sounds and work effectively even in a noisy environment. One also becomes habituated to the clothes he wears and to his own bodily sensations. These enter awareness rarely, only under special circumstances. In this sense habituation is learning to ignore recurrent external or internal stimuli that have lost novelty or meaning. Habituation develops not only in reflex response systems but in instinctive response systems as well, with the result that an animal can respond more effectively to other stimuli, such as those necessary for his survival and that of his species (Peeke, Hertz, and Gallagher, 1971). For example, a fish will defend his territory against a nonspecific intruder. Upon repeated exposure to an intruder, to whom he has no access, the fish will gradually suppress his aggressive behavior, permitting him to respond more frequently to sexually prepared females.

Besides being important in its own right, habituation is also frequently involved in more complex learning, which consists not only in acquiring new responses but also in learning to reduce errors by eliminating responses to inappropriate stimuli.

Once a response is habituated, two processes can lead to its restoration: (1) *spontaneous recovery*, which occurs as a result of withholding the habituating stimulus (Figure 6A); and (2) *dishabituation*, which occurs as a result of changing the stimulus pattern, for example, by presenting another, stronger stimulus to another pathway (Figure 6B).

With repeated stimulation of the siphon at half-minute to three-minute intervals, the gill-withdrawal reflex undergoes progressive habituation to roughly 30% of control. Typically the major decrement occurs as a result of the first five stimuli (trials). After a training session of ten trials, there is a rapid phase of recovery from habituation lasting 10 to 20 min that accounts for about 75 to 85% of reflex restoration. This is followed by a slow and highly variable return of the reflex response to its original level, often lasting many hours. But almost immediate restoration of reflex responsiveness can be obtained by presenting a single strong dishabituatory stimulus to another part of the receptive field (Figure 6B).

Relation of Habituation of the Withdrawal Reflex to Habituation of the Local Pinnule Response and to Centrally Commanded Gill Contraction Peretz (1970) has recently shown that the pinnule response also undergoes habituation. Kupfermann et al. (1971) therefore examined whether habituation of the gill-withdrawal response and of pinnule

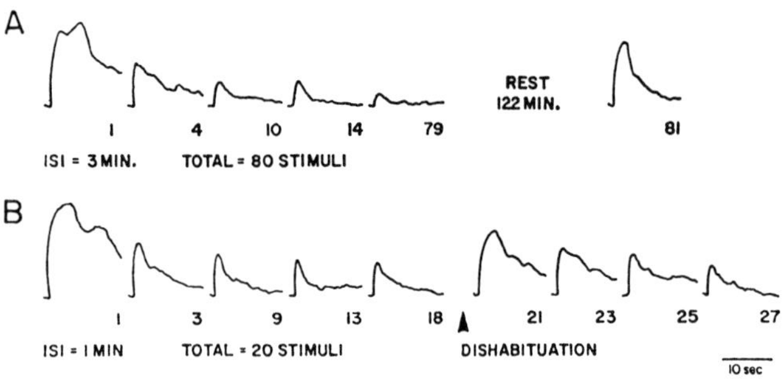

FIGURE 6 Short-term habituation and dishabituation of the gill-withdrawal reflex. Behavioral data from the intact animal (as in Figure 2B) illustrating habituation, recovery, and dishabituation. A contraction of the gill results in an upward deflection of the polygraph record (A1). With repeated stimulation at 3 min (*top*) or 1 min (*bottom*) intervals, gill response habituated to roughly 30% of control as is shown in the two separate habituation runs on the left. When recovery from habituation was tested following complete rest, without interposed stimuli, almost complete recovery occurred following 2 hr of rest (right half of A). Following rehabituation of the response (left half of B), a single strong stimulus presented to another part of the receptive field produced dishabituation (right half of B). ISI = interstimulus intervals. (From Pinsker et al., 1970.)

withdrawal are related. They found that habituation of the gill-withdrawal reflex did not affect the pinnule response and that habituation of the pinnule response did not affect the magnitude of the gill-withdrawal reflex elicited by siphon stimulation. Although one cannot rule out a small contribution from peripheral pathways to the habituation of the reflex response, the data indicate that the two behavioral modifications are independent and that habituation of the gill-withdrawal reflex is largely if not totally dependent on central pathways. Indeed the failure of generalization of habituation from one pathway to another provides further support for the independence of the central and peripheral pathways in the gill.

Similarly, Pinsker et al. (1970) examined the interaction of the reflex response and the centrally commanded contractions. They found that the centrally commanded gill contractions were of identical size before reflex habituation, during maximal response decrement, and following recovery. These experiments provide indirect evidence that habituation of the gill-withdrawal reflex is not due to muscle fatigue, as directly shown below.

Locus and Nature of the Functional Changes in the Neural Circuit of the Gill-Withdrawal Reflex During Habituation and Dishabituation The schematic drawing of the circuit of the gill-withdrawal reflex (Figure 5B2) shows that even within a simple neuronal circuit such as this, there are several possible sites (Figure 5B2: 1 to 8) for plasticity that could account for behavioral modifications.

The first question to answer was whether or not habituation involved peripheral changes, external to the CNS, either in the muscle (Figure 5B2: 2), in the sensory receptors, or in the skin (Figure 5B2: 1). The role of sensory adaptation was investigated by recording extracellularly from single afferent fibers in peripheral nerves and intracellularly from sensory neurons (Kupfermann et al., 1970; Castellucci et al., 1970; Byrne, Castellucci, and Kandel, 1973). When the skin was stimulated at intervals that produce habituation, no significant changes were found in the response of the sensory neurons. Additional evidence that changes in receptor responsiveness could not explain habituation was provided by experiments in which stimulation of the receptors was circumvented by applying a constant electrical stimulus to the afferent nerve. Under these circumstances rapid reflex habituation was still obtained (see below, Figure 7B).

The next possibility was that habituation occurred at either the neuromuscular junction or the muscle itself (Figure 5B2: 2). However, direct stimulation of the motor neurons or efferent nerves at intervals that produced habituation also did not produce significant decrement of gill contraction. Moreover the size of a directly evoked gill response produced by intracellular stimulation of a gill motor neuron was the same before and after habituation (Kupfermann et al., 1970).

Habituation must therefore result from some change within the central nervous system (Figure 5B2: 3 to 7). To determine its nature, Kupfermann et al. (1970) recorded from the major motor neurons in the intact animal (Figure 2C) during the course of habituation. They found that in the rested state, tactile stimulation of the siphon produced large and effective excitatory synaptic potentials (EPSPs) that caused repetitive discharges in the identified motor neurons that innervate the gill. When the tactile stimulus was repeated, however, the number and frequency of evoked spikes decreased (Figure 7A1). Recovery of reflex responsiveness produced either by rest (Figure 7A2) or a dishabituatory stimulus (Figure 7A3) was associated with an increase in the number and frequency of spikes in the gill motor neurons. Since the gill contraction is determined by the output of several motor neurons, the magnitude of the gill contraction was not perfectly correlated with spiking in any one motor neuron. The correlation was reasonably close, however, and a decrease of one or two spikes in the initial discharge following tactile stimulation of L7 or LD_{G1} was often associated with a measurable decrease of the gill contraction. This is consistent with the results obtained with intracellular stimulation of these cells in the same experiments where the magnitude of the gill contraction was also found to be quite sensitive to changes in spike output of the motor cells.

To determine the cellular changes underlying the alterations in firing frequency of the motor neuron, the motor cells were hyperpolarized and the changes in PSP amplitude were examined. These experiments showed that during habituation there was a progressive decrease in the amplitude of the PSPs evoked in the motor neuron by siphon stimulation that accounted for the changes in firing rate (Figure 7B1). With rest (Figure 7B2) and dishabituation (Figure 7B3) there was a restoration of the PSP amplitude (Castellucci, Pinsker, Kupfermann, and Kandel, 1970).

The decrease in the PSP during habituation was found to be due to a decrease in excitatory synaptic transmission (Figure 5B2: 7, 8) and not to a progressive increase of an underlying inhibitory postsynaptic potential (Figure 5B2: 3). Similar PSP decrement occurred when the membrane was hyperpolarized well beyond the equilibrium potential of the spontaneous IPSPs in these motor neurons. Additional evidence that IPSP potentiation does not produce the PSP decrement was provided by experiments on monosynaptic inputs discussed below. The same experiments also made it unlikely that the PSP decrement is due to presynaptic or remote inhibition.

Analysis of habituation The decrease in EPSP amplitude that occurs during habituation could result from a change either in the input resistance of the motor neuron (Figure 5B2: 6) or in the synaptic input to the motor neuron (Figure 5B2: 4, 5, 7, 8). To distinguish between these possibilities, Castellucci et al. (1970) developed a test system in which the neural circuit of the reflex could be examined in greater detail. They isolated the ganglion, with or without the siphon and the gill, and worked with it in an experimental chamber perfused with sea water (Figure 2D). To monitor the reflex output they recorded intracellularly from L7, one of the major motor neurons. To elicit the reflex response, the siphon nerve, which carries the afferent input from the siphon skin, was electrically stimulated. The complex EPSPs elicited by

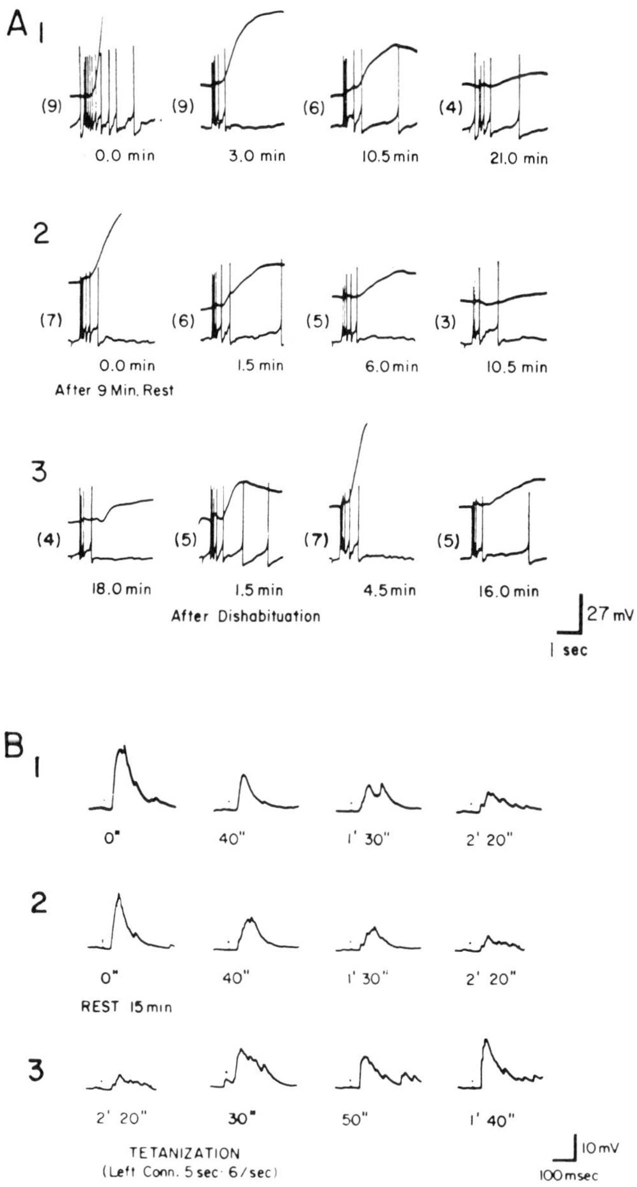

FIGURE 7 Central synaptic changes accompanying habituation, recovery and dishabituation. (A) Correlation between gill contraction and motor neuron response in a relatively intact preparation as in Figure 2C. Gill contractions (*top trace*) and simultaneous intracellular recordings from an identified motor neuron (L7) (*bottom trace*). (A1) Habituation run: Stimuli were presented every 90 sec over a period of 21 min. (A2) Partial recovery after a 9 min rest and subsequent rehabituation of the reflex. (A3) Following the last habituation trial shown in the first record of the row, a dishabituatory stimulus was introduced. Numbers in parentheses indicate numbers of spikes during first second after beginning of response. (From Kupfermann et al., 1970.) (B) Test system of the gill-withdrawal reflex in isolated ganglion as in Figure 2D. Change in complex EPSP produced in motor neuron L7 following electrical stimulation of siphon nerve at a rate of 1 per 10 sec. The membrane potential of L7 was hyperpolarized to the reversal level of the IPSP to prevent spike generation. (B1) With repeated stimulation of the siphon nerve the EPSP decreased in amplitude. (B2) It recovered with 15 min rest and then decreased again when stimulation was resumed. (B3) Tetanization (6/sec for 5 sec) of the left connective produced an immediate increase in EPSP amplitude paralleling the behavioral dishabituation. (From Schwartz et al., 1971.)

stimulating the siphon nerve resemble those produced in L7 by natural stimuli to the siphon (Figure 2B1). When the siphon nerve is stimulated repeatedly at intervals (10 sec to 2 min) that produce habituation in the whole animal, the complex PSPs decrease (Figure 7B1) and they recover their amplitude after a period of rest (Figure 7B2).

During the decrement of the EPSP no changes occurred in the input resistance of the motor neuron. These measurements are not completely conclusive because they do not rule out resistance changes at a site remote from the microelectrode in the cell body. They do, however, rule out a gross change in input resistance near the cell body and suggest that PSP alterations are more likely due to changes in the synaptic input.

A decrease in the synaptic input to the motor neuron could, in turn, be caused by an increase in central inhibition that alters the number or the firing frequency of the active afferent elements contributing to the complex EPSP (Figure 5B2: 3 or 5), or by a decrease in synaptic efficacy of individual afferent excitatory elements (Figure 5B2: 7 or 8). A demonstration of PSP decrement when a single afferent fiber is stimulated would provide an answer to this question. Castellucci et al. (1970) therefore further simplified the afferent limb of the reflex pathway by intracellular stimulation of a single mechanoreceptor neuron. Each spike in such a cell produced an elementary, presumably monosynaptic, EPSP of constant and short latency in the motor neuron (Figure 4A). When stimulated repeatedly, the changes in the magnitude of these EPSPs paralleled the habituation of the reflex; they showed decrement with repeated stimulation and recovery of their amplitude with rest (Figure 8A).

These experiments provide evidence that response decrement can occur in an excitatory monosynaptic system. Because a single sensory neuron was stimulated, the likelihood is reduced that the EPSP decrement is due to presynaptic inhibition resulting from the activation of parallel elements that act upon and inhibit the presynaptic terminals of the primary sensory neurons (Figure 5B2: 4 and 5). Rather, the findings suggest that decrement of the EPSP is the result of homosynaptic (low-frequency) depression of the excitatory synapse due either to an alteration in the mechanism of transmitter release or to a change in sensitivity of the postsynaptic receptor (Figure 5B2: 8). More recently Castellucci and Kandel (in preparation) have found that similar changes occur in the PSPs produced by the sensory neurons on the excitatory interneurons, on the inhibitory interneurons (L16), and on some motor neurons to the siphon. When two branches of the same sensory neuron, innervating different motor or interneurons, were ex-

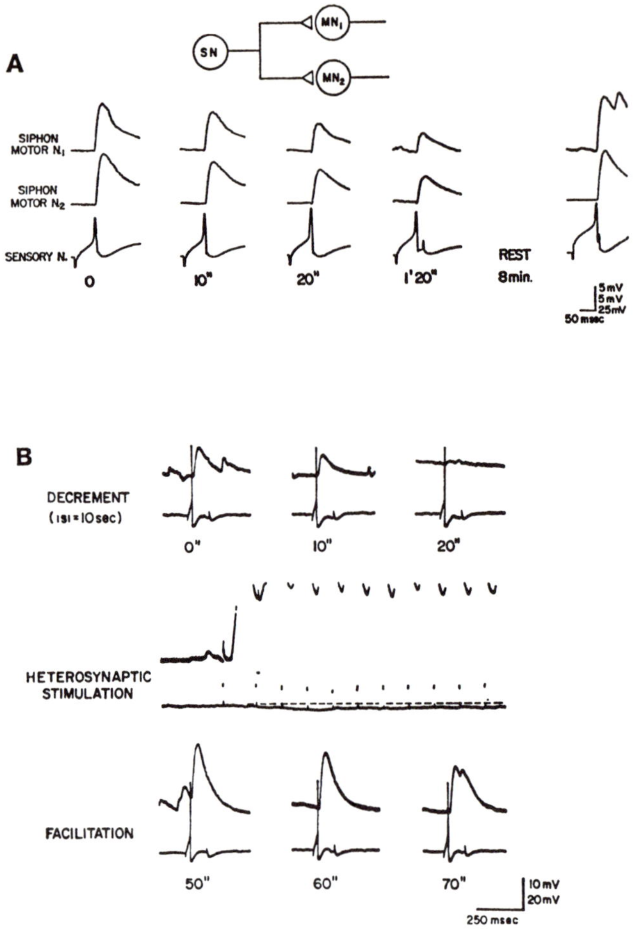

FIGURE 8 Changes in the efficacy of an elementary presumably monosynaptic connection between sensory and motor neurons due to repetitive stimulation and heterosynaptic facilitation. (A) Simultaneous recording of the EPSPs produced by repeated stimulation of one sensory neuron (interstimulus interval 10 sec) in two siphon motor neurons (MN). Note the decrement and the recovery of PSP amplitude after a rest. (From Castellucci and Kandel, in preparation.) (B) Decrement and facilitation of EPSP in the gill motor neuron L7. Intracellular stimulation of a sensory cell (lower trace of each pair) was repeated every 10 sec and produced decrement of the EPSP on L7 (top set of traces). In the middle set of traces heterosynaptic stimulation was applied to the left connective (7/sec for 5.5 sec). The heterosynaptic stimulus did not fire the sensory neuron (note the stimulus artifact in SN trace) but caused a sustained hyperpolarization in it. After the heterosynaptic stimulation (bottom set of traces) the EPSP was facilitated for several minutes. All indicated times are referred to the first stimulus (0″). The decrement illustrated is the third training session of this experiment and is therefore very rapid and profound. (From Carew, Castellucci, and Kandel, 1971.)

amined simultaneously, both showed comparable, although not always identical, decrements (Figure 8A). These results indicate that the major loci of habituation of the gill-withdrawal reflex are at the synapses made by branches of the sensory neurons on the interneurons and motor neurons responsible for the gill-withdrawal reflex. A similar locus for habituation of defensive reflexes has now been found in crayfish (Zucker, 1972) and in insects (Callec et al., 1971).

Analysis of dishabituation Castellucci et al. (1970) also examined dishabituation in the test system of the isolated ganglion and found that a strong stimulus to the pleuro-abdominal connective, equivalent to one leading to dishabituation, produced facilitation of the decremented complex EPSP (Figure 7B3). This facilitation was not accompanied by a measurable change in the input resistance of the motor neuron, nor could it be ascribed to an action on the presynaptic terminals of the sensory neurons or interneurons by spike generation in the motor neuron. Spike generation triggered by intracellular stimulation of the motor neuron produced no facilitation of the EPSP. The facilitation occurred in an elementary EPSP produced by direct stimulation of the cell body of the mechanoreceptor neuron (Figure 8B). The facilitation did not involve a change in the frequency of firing of the sensory neuron, thereby excluding post-tetanic potentiation as a mechanism for facilitation. These data suggest that the restoration of the EPSP by a dishabituatory stimulus is due to heterosynaptic facilitation (Kandel and Tauc, 1965a, 1965b).

The simplified circuit diagram of Figure 9 illustrates the locus and the mechanism for these plastic changes as suggested by Castellucci et al. (1970). Only the motor neuron (L7) on which most of the work with the elementary EPSP was done is shown. Habituation occurs as a result of repetitive stimulation of tactile receptors that leads to a homosynaptic plastic change at the indicated synapse between the afferent fiber and the motor neuron. The exact mechanism of the synaptic change is uncertain. A change in postsynaptic receptor sensitivity could not be excluded, although this mechanism seems somewhat less likely in view of the ease with which heterosynaptic facilitation occurs. By analogy with brief low-frequency depression that has now been analyzed in detail at vertebrate and crayfish neuromuscular junction (del Castillo and Katz, 1954; Dudel and Kuffler, 1961), Castellucci et al. 1970 suggested that the decrement of the elementary EPSP represents a decrease in the release of excitatory transmitter from the presynaptic terminal (see also Bruner and Tauc, 1966a and 1966b; Bruner and Kehoe, 1970). However, unlike the brief low-frequency depression evident at many synapses, those in the habituation pathway show a remarkably large and prolonged decrement. This basic difference from the usual forms of low-frequency depression requires that additional features be operative in synapses of the habituating pathway. Such factors might be a highly

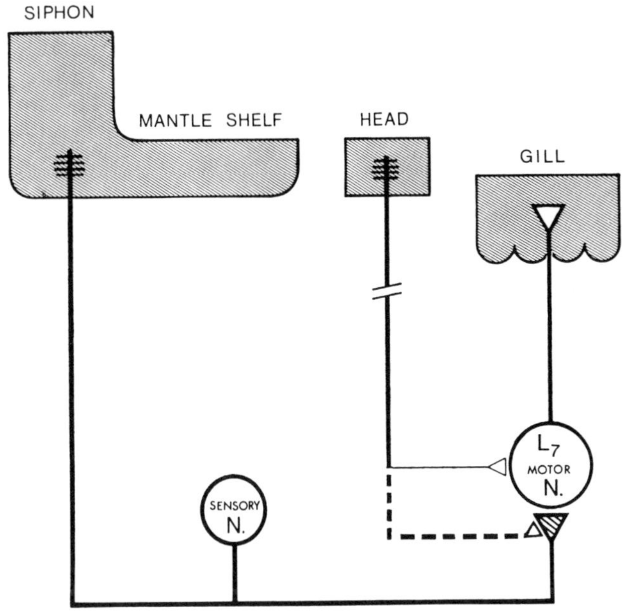

FIGURE 9 Simplified schematic diagram to indicate the postulated plastic changes in the wiring diagram of the gill reflex underlying habituation and dishabituation. See text for details. (From Castellucci et al., 1970.)

limited reservoir of immediately available transmitter substance and a slow mobilization of transmitter into this reservoir from the storage pool. Alternatively, there could be a progressive decrease in the probability of transmitter release or a decrease in the number of active presynaptic release sites.

Dishabituation occurs as a result of heterosynaptic facilitation. An attractive model for heterosynaptic facilitation is that of presynaptic facilitation at the same synapse resulting in an enhanced release of transmitter substance. Such a mechanism might operate by mobilizing transmitter substance from the storage pool to the immediately available transmitter reservoir, by increasing the probability of releasing transmitter, or by increasing the number of active release sites. Since the elementary PSPs in the presumed monosynaptic pathways are quite large, changes in their efficacy may account fully for at least the early component of habituation and dishabituation of the gill response in *Aplysia*.

This analysis demonstrates that habituation and dishabituation of this reflex involves plastic changes in the excitatory transmission of previously existing connections. No fundamental changes occurred in the wiring diagram; no new connection appeared and no existing connections disappeared. Instead, the functional effectiveness of certain previously existing connections was changed. The synapses between the sensory neuron and inter- and motor-neuron are endowed with remarkable plastic properties so that transmission across the synapse is greatly decreased during habituation and recovers only slowly after rest; it is restored immediately, however, by a dishabituating stimulus. These results are therefore consistent with the idea that genetic and developmental processes determine the properties of the individual cells and the anatomical interconnections between them. These processes leave unspecified the degree of effectiveness of certain of these connections. Environmental factors can play upon these plastic capabilities such as short-term learning to produce behavioral events.

Short-Term Habituation and Dishabituation in the Absence of Protein Synthesis Once a behavioral modification has been specified in cellular terms, it should be possible to bring biochemical techniques to bear on the analysis of molecular mechanisms of learning. As a start, Schwartz, Castellucci and Kandel (1971) examined the action on the neuronal correlates of habituation and dishabituation of three antibiotics (anisomycin, sparsomycin and pactamycin) that inhibit protein synthesis in the abdominal ganglion by more than 95%. The effect of these antibiotics was studied in the isolated ganglion using the test system of the gill-withdrawal reflex (Figure 2D). Repeated stimulation was applied to the siphon nerve, and the neuronal correlates of habituation and dishabituation were monitored in the absence or in the presence of anisomycin. Neither the change in synaptic efficacy associated with habituation or that associated with dishabituation were found to be affected by prior incubation in anisomycin for up to 6 hr. Longer periods of incubation were not examined.

Although long-term habituation may depend on new protein synthesis, these results indicate that short-term habituation and dishabituation do not, nor do they depend on the synthesis of proteins that have remarkably fast turn-over rates. This result is consistent with experiments in vertebrates, which indicates that new protein synthesis is not required for short-term learning (see for example, Agranoff, 1967; Barondes, 1970). These findings also draw attention to a need for biochemical models other than alterations in macromolecular synthesis to explain the mechanisms underlying short-term neuronal plasticity. As I have mentioned above, the synaptic changes associated with habituation and dishabituation might be due to prolonged alterations in transmitter release. Alternatively, but perhaps less likely, one or both of these processes could reflect a change in receptor sensitivity. Alterations in molecular conformation might not be expected to persist for long periods of time, although molecular changes lasting for several minutes have been observed (see Frieden, 1970). More likely, the biochemical mechanisms underlying these short-term plastic changes are composed of a series of sequential reactions that result in a new distribution of transmitter substance or its availability. Mechanisms involving cyclic 3′, 5′ AMP might serve as one example of a series of reactions that result in transient enhancement in the activity of a critical enzyme system (Rall and Gilman, 1970; Rasmussen, 1970). A pathway of this kind might trigger the mobilization of transmitter from one compartment (a long-term store) to another (an immediately releasable store) or might control the number and availability of release sites. Several recent reports of altered synaptic activity might reasonably be explained by this mechanism (Dudel, 1965; Goldberg and Singer, 1969; Kuba, 1970). Thus, sequential reactions that include the formation of degradable small molecules but that do not involve the production of new structural, receptor, or enzymatic components, could account at least for short-term plastic changes.

Whether or not new protein synthesis is essential for the transition to long-term memory could in principle also be examined in simple systems.

Interrelationships between different behavioral modifications

Cellular studies can also help clarify questions about the relationship between different behavioral modifications. Two examples are considered here: (1) the relationship of habituation to dishabituation, and (2) the relationship of short- to long-term memory.

Relationship of Habituation to Dishabituation There is disagreement among students of behavior as to whether dishabituation is a reversal of habituation (Pavlov, 1927; Humphrey, 1930, 1933; Konorski, 1967; Sokolov, 1963; Wickelgren, 1967; Wall, 1970) or a different, and in some ways independent, facilitatory process superimposed upon habituation (Sharpless and Jasper, 1956; Spencer, Thompson, and Neilson, 1966; Groves and Thompson, 1970). This question was examined by Carew, Castellucci, and Kandel (1971), at both the behavioral and neurophysiological levels, using another property of the gill-withdrawal reflex, the lack of generalization of habituation from one pathway to another (Figure 10A).

The receptive field of the gill-withdrawal reflex consists of the siphon and the edge of the mantle shelf that contains the purple gland (Figure 10A1). The anterior portion of the mantle shelf and the purple gland are innervated by a branch of the branchial nerve. The siphon and the posterior third of the purple gland and mantle shelf are innervated by the siphon nerve (Figures

10A1, 10A2). The siphon and the anterior third of the mantle shelf (purple gland) therefore provide two limited distinct afferent pathways for a common motor response. In intact animals habituation of the reflex response via one pathway does not alter responsiveness via the other pathway. Similarly, decrement of the PSPs produced by repeated electrical stimulation of one pathway does not affect PSP responsiveness from the other pathway (Figures 10A2, 10A3).

To examine the relationship of dishabituation to habituation, Carew, Castellucci, and Kandel (1971) compared the effects of a common "dishabituatory" stimulus on both habituated and nonhabituated responses using these two different reflex pathways. If the dishabituation is due to a reversal of habituation, the "dishabituatory" stimulus should facilitate only the habituated pathway and bring it up to its original value. If dishabituation is a superimposed facilitation (sensitization), then a "dishabituatory" stimulus might facilitate a nonhabituated response. In addition, the habituated responses might be facilitated *beyond* their control value.

In behavioral experiments a single test stimulus was presented to either the siphon or the anterior third of the purple gland of an intact restrained animal. The reflex was then habituated by repeated stimulation of the other pathway. Following a second test stimulus to the nonhabituated pathway, a strong tactile stimulus was presented to the head or neck region of the animal. Dishabituation of the habituated pathway was observed in every preparation and was occasionally *larger* than the initial control value. Sensitization of the nonhabituated pathway was only found in one-third of the animals but in 5 of 6 cases where the neck stimulus produced sensitization, it also produced dishabituation. In the sixth case dishabituation could not be examined. As we shall

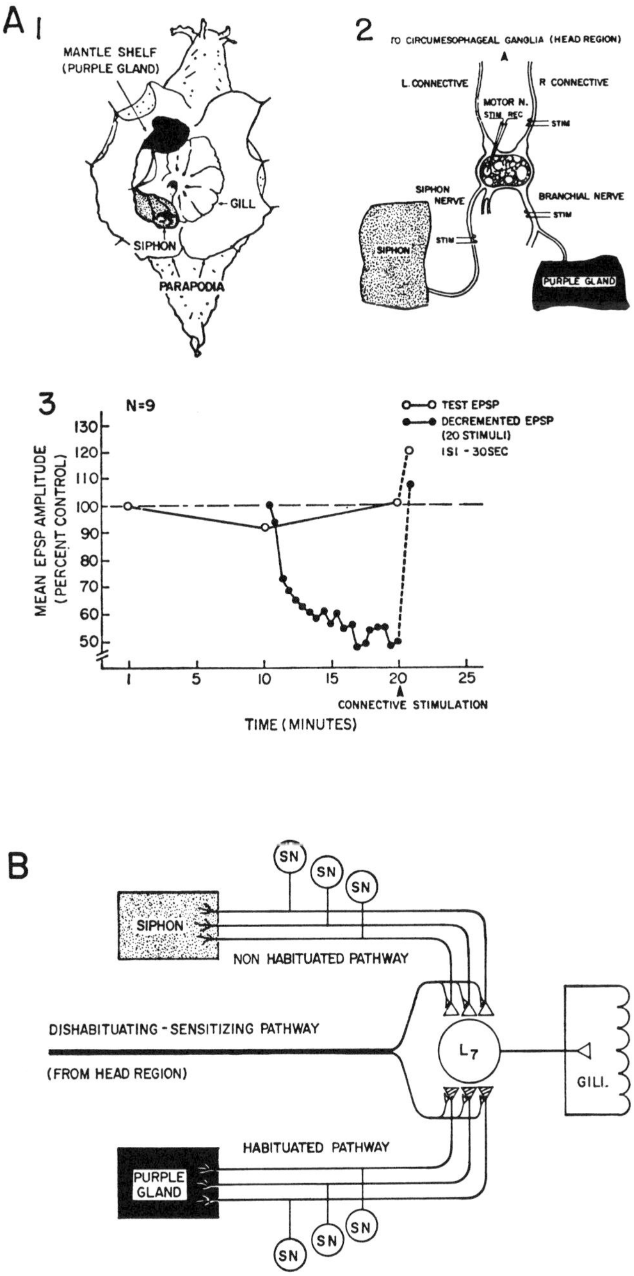

FIGURE 10 Relation of habituation of the gill-withdrawal reflex to dishabituation and sensitization. (A) Behavioral and cellular neurophysiological preparations. (A1) Dorsal view of an intact *Aplysia*. The parapodia and mantle shelf have been retracted to reveal the gill. The anterior part of the mantle shelf and purple gland are indicated by solid black lines. The siphon and the posterior part of the mantle shelf are stippled. The two sites have a separate innervation and were used as independent reflex inputs for gill withdrawal. (A2) Diagram illustrating test system in isolated ganglion. In the test system the branchial nerve, which innervates the anterior part of the mantle shelf and purple gland, or the siphon nerve, which innervates the posterior part of the purple gland, and siphon were electrically stimulated. Stimulation of the right or left connective provided stimuli for heterosynaptic facilitation. (A3) Summary graph of 9 runs from 4 different preparations showing absence of generalization of EPSP decrement between decremented and test inputs to the motor neuron (L7). Following a single train of stimuli (6 per sec for 6 sec) to the connective (connective stimulation ↑), facilitated both decremented and nondecremented responses. (B) Schematic diagram illustrating the difference in spatial extent of the pathways mediating habituation (shaded synapses) and sensitization (or dishabituation). Diagram explains the lack of generalization of habituation as well as the evident generalization of sensitization (dishabituation). The model postulates that the sensitizing pathway (which is not necessarily monosynaptic) mediates presynaptic facilitation on the synapse between the primary sensory neurons (SN) and the motor neuron L7 (here used as a model for the entire reflex). (From Carew, Castellucci, and Kandel, 1971.)

see below (Figure 13), unrestrained animals showed profound sensitization (Pinsker, Carew and Kandel, 1972), and its absence in restrained animals may have resulted from sensitization caused by the restraint.

In cellular neurophysiological experiments, Carew et al. (1971) examined how the neuronal correlates of dishabituation relate to those of sensitization, using the test system of the isolated ganglion. They stimulated either the branchial or siphon nerve repeatedly and produced decrement of the EPSP. They then examined the effect of a heterosynaptic stimulus, applied to a connective, on the amplitude of the decremented EPSP produced by the previously stimulated pathway and on the amplitude of the nondecremented EPSP produced by the pathway not previously stimulated. They found that the decremented EPSP was invariably facilitated and in 70% of the cases the facilitated EPSP was larger than the initial (nondecremented) control. The same stimulus to the connective also facilitated the nondecremented EPSP in 80% of the cases (Figure 10A3). Both decremented and nondecremented PSPs showed similar increases (about 120%) compared to their *initial* controls. The decremented EPSPs obviously showed proportionately more facilitation (224%) when the last observed (decremented) response was used as control, instead of the first of the series.

Thus, in behavioral experiments, the same strong stimulus that produced dishabituation of a habituated pathway was also capable of producing sensitization of a nonhabituated pathway, at least some of the time. In the neurophysiological experiments the same strong stimulus that produced facilitation of a decremented EPSP usually also produced facilitation of a nondecremented EPSP. Taken together, these two sets of data support the notion that dishabituation of the gill-withdrawal reflex is not simply the removal of habituation but is an independent facilitation. Dishabituation is thus a special case of sensitization (Spencer, Thompson, and Neilson, 1966) that differs from it only in involving a previously habituated response. The neuronal correlates of habituation and dishabituation (sensitization) are thus not mirror image processes but reflect two separate regulatory mechanisms acting on a common set of synapses. Indeed, these two processes have different spatial distributions (Figure 10B). Whereas habituation is limited to the stimulated pathway, sensitization has a more widespread distribution involving both stimulated and unstimulated pathways. The difference in the extent of the pathways mediating habituation and sensitization (dishabituation) explains the lack of generalization of habituation as well as the evident generalization of sensitization to nonhabituated pathways.

Relationship of Short- to Long-Term Habituation

A particularly important current problem in behavioral psychology is the relation of short- to long-term memory. Experiments that interfere with normal brain function, such as inhibition of protein synthesis or electroconvulsive shock, suggest that short- and long-term memory are distinct. Short-term memory is thought to be impaired by electroconvulsive shock whereas long-term memory is obliterated by inhibition of protein synthesis. (For review, see Agranoff, 1967; Barondes, 1970). These experiments support the dual-trace theory of memory advocated by Hebb (1949), which postulates that a short-term "holding" process somehow leads to long-term storage. However, the interpretation of the electroconvulsive shock and protein inhibition experiments is not clear cut (Weiskrantz, 1970). To determine whether long-term memory is a distinct process or an extension of the short-term process requires a system in which these questions can be examined on the cellular level.

Toward this end, Carew, Pinsker, and Kandel (1972) have developed a training procedure for studying long-term habituation that permits a mechanistic analysis of the transition from short- to long-term habituation. As we have seen, ten habituation trials in one session lead to habituation that is largely dissipated several hours later. To examine long-term habituation, one cannot work on the restrained animal, because animals do not survive for several days if restrained. Carew et al. (1972) thus studied unrestrained animals using the siphon component instead of the gill component of the defensive reflex as an index of reflex withdrawal (Figure 1B). When habituation training (10 trials/day) is repeated daily for 4 days, habituation of the reflex response builds up progressively across days so that habituation occurs more rapidly on each subsequent day. Thus on day 5 the median net duration of reflex response during ten trials is only 20% of its duration on day 1 (Figures 11A1, 11A2). The habituation is long lasting and persists unchanged for a week, recovering only partially after three weeks (Figures 11A1, 11A2). This makes it possible to use this system as a potential model for studying the acquisition of long-term memory.

Whereas the siphon component of the withdrawal reflex offers the advantage that it can be studied in the freely moving animal, it has potential disadvantages. Unlike the gill-withdrawal component, which is centrally mediated, the siphon withdrawal component is known to involve some contribution from the peripheral nerve net (Kupfermann and Kesselman, 1968; Lukowiak and Jacklet, 1972; Newby, 1972), because, to elicit siphon withdrawal, the stimulus is applied to the siphon itself, which optimizes the recruitment of peripherally mediated responses (Bethe, 1903). To determine the relative contribution of peripheral and central components of the siphon withdrawal in the intact animal, Pinsker, Carew, and Kandel (1973) examined siphon withdrawal both in normal animals and in animals from which the abdominal ganglion had been surgically removed. They found that whereas normal (unhabituated) animals routinely withdrew the siphon beyond the parapodia (Figure 1B2), deganglionated animals did not and gave only very slight responses.

To obtain an independent evaluation of the central contribution, Carew et al. (1972) undertook another series of experiments, this time on the gill component of the reflex, in order to ascertain whether the type of siphon stimulation that produced long-term habituation of the siphon component of the defensive reflex also

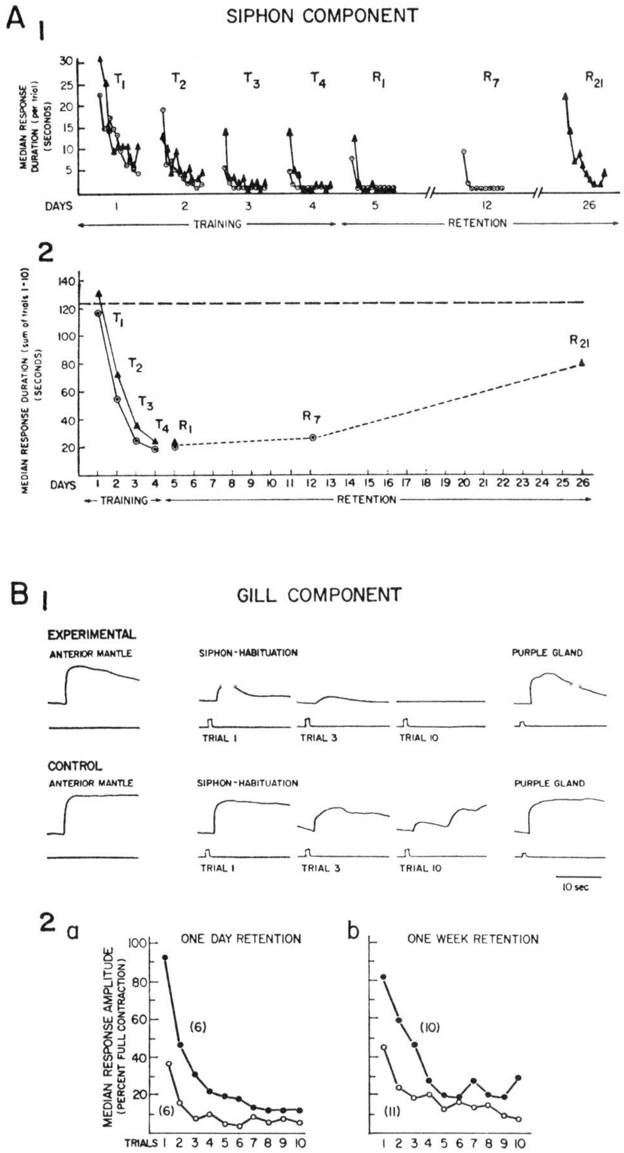

FIGURE 11 Long-term habituation of both siphon and gill components of the defensive withdrawal reflex. (A) Long-term habituation of siphon component. (A_1) Build-up of habituation during training for 4 days (T1 to T4) and retention after 24 hr (R1), 1 week (R7), and 3 weeks (R21). Data from three experiments (n = 19) are presented: Two independent, identical replications in which retention was tested at 24 hr and 1 week have been pooled (⊙—⊙); in the third experiment (n = 14), retention was tested at 24 hr and 3 weeks (△—△). Each data point is the median duration of siphon withdrawal for each of ten habituation trials. (Parallel control data (n = 20, n = 14) are presented in Carew et al., 1971. Figure 1.) (A2) Time course of habituation. Habituation within each daily session is expressed as a single score, the sum of ten trials (the net amount of time of siphon withdrawal during the entire habituation training session). The upper dashed line indicates control habituation (day 1 of training). Compare retention tested at 24 hr (day 5) and 1 week, day 12 (⊙—⊙) and retention at 24 hr (day 5) and 3 weeks, day 26 (△—△) with control (day 1) habituation. (B) Long-term habituation of gill component. (B1) Gill-withdrawal reflexes were recorded with a photocell. One week previously, experimental animals had shown significant 24-hr retention of habituation of siphon withdrawal as compared to controls. Retention of habituation of gill withdrawal (produced by the previous siphon habituation training) was measured 7 days later in restrained animals. A single test gill contraction was first produced by vigorous tactile stimulation of the anterior mantle region (first column). After a brief period of rest, habituation of gill withdrawal was produced by repetitive siphon stimulation with a jet of sea water (ten trials; interstimulus interval, 30 sec), and this was followed by another single test stimulus to the purple gland. Anterior mantle or purple gland stimulation produced comparable contractions in both experimental and control animals. However, siphon stimulation produced a significantly reduced initial gill withdrawal in experimental than in control animals (compare trials 1, 3, and 10 of both records). Time calibration, 10 sec. (B2) Comparison of experimental and control habituation of gill withdrawal at 1 day and 1 week. Median amplitude of gill responses expressed as a percentage of a full contraction. The number of animals in each group is indicated in parentheses. (B2a) Gill withdrawal 24 hr after siphon habituation training. Experimental animals (●—●) exhibited significantly greater habituation ($P < 0.001$) of gill withdrawal (sum of trials 1 to 10) than controls (○—○) and were significantly lower than controls on 9 out of 10 trials. (B2b) Gill withdrawal 7 days after siphon habituation training. Experimental animals again exhibited significantly greater habituation ($P < 0.001$) and were significantly lower than controls on 8 out of 10 trials. These data indicate that stimuli that produce long-term habituation of siphon withdrawal also produce long-term habituation of gill withdrawal. (From Carew, Pinsker, and Kandel, 1972.)

produced long-term habituation of the gill component. Either 1 or 7 days after the 4-day habituation training sessions in freely moving animals, experimental animals were mixed with controls, and the gill-withdrawal reflex of both groups was measured (by a blind procedure) with the animals restrained and a photocell placed under the gill (Figure 2B). In the testing procedure, as in the training procedure, habituation was produced by ten trials of siphon stimulation. Both 1-day and 7-day experimental animals exhibited significantly greater habituation of gill withdrawal than controls (Figure 11B), indicating that repeated siphon stimulation produces long-term habituation not only of the siphon component of this reflex but also of the gill component.

Whereas the reflex responsiveness to siphon stimulation was significantly reduced in experimental animals, there was no statistical difference between gill-withdrawal reflexes produced by purple gland or anterior mantle shelf stimulation in both experimental and control animals (Figure 11B). These findings illustrate that, like short-term habituation, long-term habituation does not generalize from the siphon to nonstimulated parts of the receptive field; it is restricted specifically to the stimulated afferent pathway.

Recently Carew and Kandel (1973) have simplified the training procedure for long-term habituation by presenting the four spaced training sessions within one day, separated from each other by only $1\frac{1}{2}$ hr. This shortened spaced training procedure still leads to long-term habituation and has the advantage of making it possible to study the cellular mechanisms of acquisition and even of retention of the long-term process. In experiments with the isolated ganglion test system, stimulation of an afferent nerve with the same temporal patterning as in the behavioral experiments produced a progressive decrease in the complex EPSP that persisted for at least 24 hr. These changes in the complex EPSP look similar to the changes that accompany the short-term habituation. However, changes in the amplitude of the complex EPSP can be caused by several different mechanisms. Whether or not the long-term process is indeed an extension of the short-term one will therefore require further analysis.

RELATION OF LONG-TERM HABITUATION TO MORE COMPLEX LEARNING The kinetics and time course of long-term habituation are interesting because they resemble certain apsects of higher learning found in vertebrates and man. For example, when a human subject is asked to tap a Morse code key and hold it down for 0.7 sec, his performance improves with repeated trials (Figure 12A). Although a comparison of a few parametric features of human and invertebrate behavior is by itself not very meaningful, it is interesting to note that in *Aplysia*, as in human learning, there is a slight "forgetting" between the last performance of one day and the first performance the next day, despite the progressive improvement over days (Figure 12B).

Since, in these parametric properties, long-term habituation in *Aplysia* bears at least a superficial resemblance to behavioral modifications characteristic of vertebrates, Carew, Pinsker and Kandel (1972) looked for other features shared by long-term habituation and more complex learning. In most types of complex learning, temporally spaced training usually produces better learning than massed training (Woodworth and Schlosberg, 1954). Carew et al. therefore compared a spaced-training group (four training sessions of ten habituation trials each, separated by anywhere from 1.5 to 24 hr) with a massed-training group (one training session consisting of 40 consecutive habituation trials). Despite the fact that both groups had received the same number of training trials, animals receiving spaced training exhibited significantly greater habituation one day and one week later than did those receiving massed training (Figures 12B1 to 12B4). These data indicated that spacing habituation training by even as much as one hour is much more effective in producing long-term habituation than massing the habituation training.

Thus, despite its simplicity, habituation of gill and siphon withdrawal in *Aplysia* shows a number of interesting parallels to the complex learning of vertebrates. It not only provides an instructive paradigm for studying the neural mechanisms of short- and long-term behavioral modifications but it may also be useful for examining the mechanisms of pattern sensitivity in behavioral modifications. In particular it would be interesting to know whether the pattern of stimulation is the essential feature that is responsible for the transition from short- to long-term memory. Studies along these lines could specify how long-term memory is established and how it relates to the short-term process.

Summary and perspectives

The studies that I have outlined here and parallel ones that are now being carried out with arthropods and insects (Zucker, 1972; Callec et al., 1971) do not, as yet, increase understanding of the neural mechanisms of behavior and of learning. These studies involve relatively simple behavioral modifications in simple animals. Only the merest beginnings have been made.

Moreover, although we can now specify the locus of the neural change during short-term habituation, as in

Aplysia, and know that the critical change results from an alteration in synaptic transmission, we still have only a superficial understanding of the detailed mechanisms of the synaptic change. To obtain more meaningful insights into these mechanisms, we will need more extensive electrophysiological analysis of synaptic transmission at the critical synapses between the sensory neurons and the central neurons they innervate. In addition, morphological techniques for studying the fine structure of these synapses are needed.

If these techniques can be developed, however, it may become possible to analyze the mechanisms of more complex behaviors and more interesting instances of behavioral modifications. In addition, these preparations may ultimately be useful for studying the cellular mechanisms of behavioral abnormalities. For example, habituation occurs readily in a safe environment where an *Aplysia* learns quickly to ignore a novel but innocuous stimulus that is repeatedly presented. But animals cannot afford to habituate their withdrawal reflexes readily in a hostile environment. Pinsker, Carew, and Kandel (1973) have found that animals do not readily habituate even to an innocuous siphon stimulus if they have previously received noxious stimulation to the head. Animals receiving 2 such stimuli a day for 10 days become highly sensitized and show reflex responsiveness that differs radically from that of a normal animal (Figure 13). Animals so treated live in a dangerous environment and show the reflex behavior of an overly responsive or aroused animal. Particularly interesting is the finding that the heightened responsiveness persists for many days *after* the noxious stimulation has stopped. Although the heightened responsiveness was appropriate in the dangerous environment, it is quite inappropriate for the neutral environment in which the animal now again lives. In so far as an animal's responsiveness over the long term is less appropriately related to the immediate stimulus that elicits it than it is to certain moments in its past history, the animal can be thought of as responding inappropriately, or abnormally, to the demands of its current environment. Thus, as we gain a better understanding of the learning process, we might also be able to develop animal model systems that may permit us insights into certain behavioral abnormalities that result from learning.

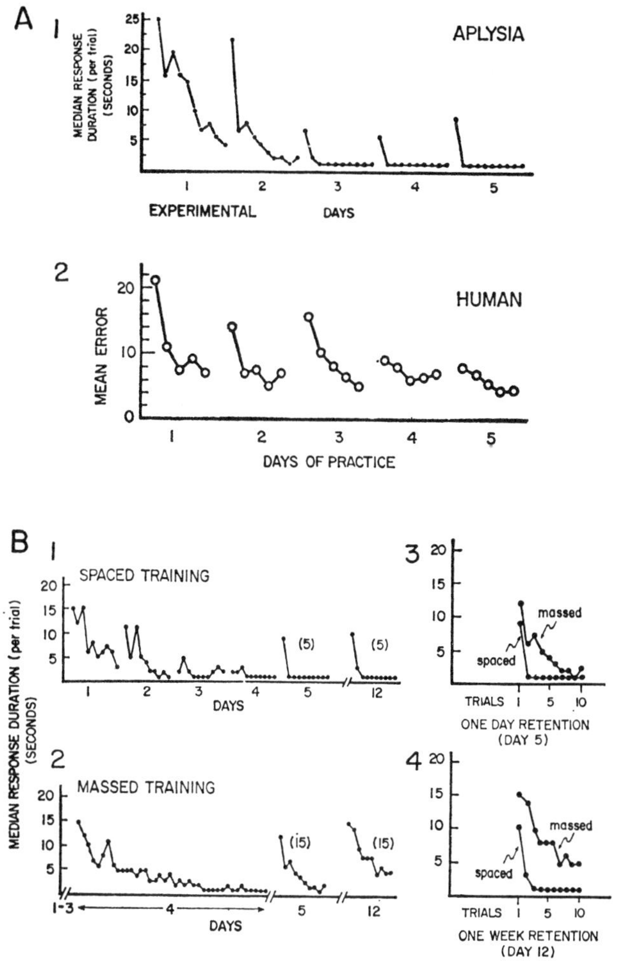

FIGURE 12 Comparison of *Aplysia* habituation to higher order behavioral modifications. (A) Comparison of habituation in *Aplysia* (A1) to human learning (A2). The human subject was asked to depress a Morse key for a duration of 0.7 sec. Subject's error from the correct duration was shown to him after each attempt providing immediate feedback. As in the *Aplysia* experiment 10 daily trials were given but at 12-sec intervals instead of 30-sec intervals. The mean error of 10 subjects for 2 successive trials are plotted. The data in *Aplysia* are taken from one of the experiments (⊙—⊙) illustrated in Figure 11A1. The human data are replotted from MacPherson, Dees, and Grindley, 1949. (B) Comparison of spaced (B1) with massed (B2) habituation training. Two groups of experimental animals were given either 4 days of habituation training (10 trials per day, spaced training) or 1 day of habituation training (40 trials, massed training). Both groups were tested for retention after 24 hr (day 5) and 1 week (day 12). The spaced training group (B1) was significantly lower than the massed-training group (B2) at both 24 hr ($p < 0.01$) and 1 week ($p < 0.01$), despite the fact that both groups had received the same number of training trials. The massed-training group was not significantly different from unstimulated control in either retention test. In the 1 week retention test (day 12) the massed training group was no longer significantly lower than their initial performance (day 4, trials 1 to 10) indicating that this group showed no retention of training after 1 week while the spaced-training group still exhibited significant retention of habituation. Number of animals in each group is indicated in parentheses. (B3 and B4.) Comparison of spaced to massed habituation on each retention day. (From Carew, Pinsker, and Kandel, 1972.)

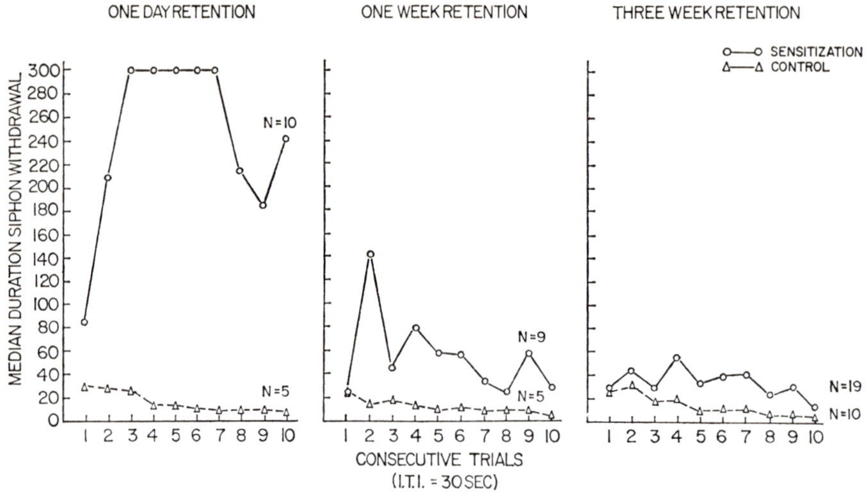

FIGURE 13 Long-term sensitization. Comparison of control animals (N=10) who received no prior training (△—△) to experimental (N=19) animals (○—○) who had received two noxious stimuli per day for 10 days (sensitization) training prior to the first day of retention. The experimental and control groups were each divided into two after training was completed. One experimental and control group was examined for one day retention, the other two groups for one week retention. The two experimental and control groups were again combined for the 3 week retention tests. On test days (1 day, 1 week, and 3 weeks after sensitization training), both control and sensitized animals received a series of ten weak tactile stimuli to the siphon by means of a jet of sea water applied by a Water Pik. The experimental animals showed an increased response, and their habituation curve had different kinetics than that of the controls showing a buildup (particularly on 1 day and 1 week retention tests) rather than the usual negatively accelerating decrement. The flat peak of the sensitization group on the one-day retention test results from the fact that more than half of the animals exceeded the 300 sec limit on those trials.

ACKNOWLEDGMENTS I thank Drs. Vincent Castellucci and Irving Kupfermann for their helpful comments on an earlier draft of this manuscript and Kathrin Hilten for her usual expert help with the figures. I am supported by a Career Scientist Award from NIMH #MH 18558-06 and the work of my laboratory is supported by grants NS 09261-03 and NIMH 19795-02.

REFERENCES

AGRANOFF, B. W., 1967. Agents that block memory. In *The Neurosciences*, G. C. Quarton, T. Melnechuk, and F. O. Schmitt, eds. New York: Rockefeller University Press, pp. 756–764.

ARVANITAKI, A., and S. H. TCHOU, 1942. Les lois de la croissance relative individuelle des cellules nerveuses chez l'*Aplysie*. *Bull. Histol. Appl. Tech. Microscop.* 19:244–256.

ARVANITAKI, A., and N. CHALAZONITIS, 1958. Configurations modales de l'activité propres à différents neurons d'un même centre. *J. Physiol.* (*Paris*) 50:122–125.

BARONDES, S. H., 1970. Multiple steps in the biology of memory. In *The Neurosciences*: *Second Study Program*, F. O. Schmitt, ed. New York: Rockefeller University Press, pp. 272–278.

BAUMGARTEN, R. J. VON, 1970. Plasticity in the nervous system at the unitary level. In *The Neurosciences: Second Study Program*, F. O. Schmitt, ed. New York: Rockefeller University Press, pp. 260–271.

BETHE, A., 1903. *Allgemeine Anatomie und Physiologie des Nervensystems*. Leipzig: Thieme.

BRUNER, J., and J. KEHOE, 1970. Long term decrements in the efficacy of synaptic transmission of molluscs and crustaceans. In *Short-Term Changes in Neural Activity and Behavior*, G. Horn and R. Hinde, eds. London: Cambridge University Press, pp. 323–359.

BRUNER, J., and L. TAUC, 1966a. Habituation at the synaptic level in *Aplysia*. *Nature* (*Lond.*) 210:37–39.

BRUNER, J., and L. TAUC, 1966b. Long-lasting phenomena in the molluscan nervous system. *Symp. Soc. Exp. Biol.* 20:457–475.

BULLOCK, T. H., and G. A. HORRIDGE, 1965. *Structure and Function in the Nervous Systems of Invertebrates*. San Francisco: W. H. Freeman.

BYRNE, J., V. CASTELLUCCI, and E. R. KANDEL, 1973. Receptive fields and response properties of mechanoreceptor neurons in the siphon skin of *Aplysia*. (In preparation.)

CALLEC, J. J., J. C. GUILLET, Y. PICHON, and J. BOISTEL, 1971. Further studies on synaptic transmission in insects. II. Relations between sensory information and its synaptic integration at the level of a single giant axon in the cockroach. *J. Exp. Biol.* 55:123–149.

CAREW, T. J., V. F. CASTELLUCCI, and E. R. KANDEL, 1971. An analysis of dishabituation and sensitization of the gill-withdrawal reflex in *Aplysia*. *Intern. J. Neuroscience*. 2:79–98.

CAREW, T. J., and E. R. KANDEL, 1973. Rapid acquisition of long-term habituation: Behavioral and cellular neurophysiological correlation. (In preparation.)

CAREW, T. J., H. M. PINSKER, and E. R. KANDEL, 1972. Long-term habituation of a defensive withdrawal reflex in *Aplysia*. *Science* 175:451–454.

CAREW, T. J., H. PINSKER, K. RUBINSON, J. H. SCHWARTZ, and E. R. KANDEL, 1973. Physiological and biochemical properties of neuromuscular transmission between identified motor neurons and gill muscle in *Aplysia*. (In preparation.)

CAREW, T. J., J. H. SCHWARTZ, and E. R. KANDEL, 1972. Innervation of *Aplysia* gill muscle fibers by two identified excitation motor neurons using different chemical transmitters. *Physiologist* 15(3):100.

Castellucci, V., H. Pinsker, I. Kupfermann, and E. R. Kandel, 1970. Neuronal mechanisms of habituation and dishabituation of the gill-withdrawal reflex in *Aplysia. Science* 167:1745–1748.

del Castillo, J., and B. Katz, 1954. The effect of magnesium on the activity of motor nerve endings. *J. Physiol.* (*Lond.*) 124: 553–559.

Diamond, J., 1971. The Mauthner Cell. In *Fish Physiology*, Vol. 5, W. S. Hoar and D. J. Randall, eds. New York: Academic Press, pp. 265–346.

Dudel, J., 1965. Facilitatory effects of 5-hydroxy-tryptamine on the crayfish neuromuscular junction. *Arch. Exptl. Pathol. Pharmakol.* 249:515–528.

Dudel, J., and S. W. Kuffler, 1961. Mechanism of facilitation at the crayfish neuromuscular junction. *J. Physiol.* (*Lond.*) 155:530–542.

Eales, N. B., 1921. *Aplysia. Proc. Trans. Liverpool Biol. Soc. Mem.* 35:183–266.

Eccles, J. C., 1953. *The Neurophysiological Basis of Mind.* Oxford: Clarendon Press.

Frazier, W. T., E. R. Kandel, I. Kupfermann, R. Waziri, and R. E. Coggeshall, 1967. Morphological and functional properties of identified neurons in the abdominal ganglion of *Aplysia californica. J. Neurophysiol.* 30:1288–1351.

Frazier, W. T., R. Waziri, and E. R. Kandel, 1965. Alterations in the frequency of spontaneous activity in *Aplysia* neurons with contingent and non-contingent nerve stimulation. *Fed. Proc.* 24(2171):522.

Frieden, C., 1970. Kinetic aspects of regulation of metabolic processes. The hysteretic enzyme concept. *J. Biol. Chem.* 245: 5788–5799.

Gardner, D., 1971. Bilateral symmetry and interneuronal organization in the buccal ganglia of *Aplysia. Science* 173: 550–553.

Gardner, D., and E. R. Kandel, 1972. Diphasic postsynaptic potential: A chemical synapse capable of mediating conjoint excitation and inhibition. *Science* 176:675–678.

Gaze, R. M., and M. J. Keating, 1972. The visual system and "neuronal specificity." *Nature* (*Lond.*) 237:375–378.

Giller, Jr., E., and J. H. Schwartz, 1968. Choline acetyltransferase: Regional distribution in the abdominal ganglion of *Aplysia. Science* 161:908–911.

Giller, Jr., E., and J. H. Schwartz, 1971a. Choline acetyltransferase in identified neurons of abdominal ganglion of *Aplysia californica. J. Neurophysiol.* 34:93–107.

Giller, Jr., E., and J. H. Schwartz, 1971b. Acetylcholinesterase in identified neurons of abdominal ganglion of *Aplysia californica. J. Neurophysiol.* 34:108–115.

Goldberg, A. L., and J. J. Singer, 1969. Evidence for a role of cyclic AMP in neuromuscular transmission. *Proc. Natl. Acad. Sci. USA* 64:134–141.

Groves, P. M., and R. F. Thompson, 1970. Habituation: A dual-process theory. *Psychol. Rev.* 77(5):419–450.

Hebb, D. O., 1949. *The Organization of Behavior.* New York: John Wiley & Sons.

Hinde, R. A., 1970. *Animal Behavior: A Synthesis of Ethology and Comparative Psychology.* (2nd edition), New York: McGraw-Hill.

Hubel, D. H., and T. N. Wiesel, 1965. Binocular interaction in striate cortex of kittens reared with artificial squint. *J, Neurophysiol.* 28:1041–1059.

Hughes, J. R., E. V. Evarts, and W. H. Marshall, 1956. Post-tetanic potentiation in the visual system of cats. *Am. J. Physiol.* 186:483–487.

Humphrey, G., 1930. Le Chatelier's rule and the problem of habituation and dishabituation in *Helix albolabris. Psychol. Forsch.* 13:113–127.

Humphrey, G., 1933. *The Nature of Learning in its Relation to Living Systems.* New York: Harcourt, Brace.

Kandel, E. R., 1967. Cellular studies of learning. In *The Neurosciences*, G. C. Quarton, T. Melnechuk, and F. O. Schmitt, eds. New York: Rockefeller University Press, pp. 666–689.

Kandel, E. R., 1968. Dale's principle and the functional specificity of neurons. In *Psychopharmacology: A Review of Progress* 1957–1967, D. E. Efron, ed. Public Health Service Publ. No. 1836. U.S. Govt. Printing Office, pp. 385–398.

Kandel, E. R., W. T. Frazier, R. Waziri, and R. E. Coggeshall, 1967. Direct and common connections among identified neurons in *Aplysia. J. Neurophysiol.* 30:1352–1376.

Kandel, E. R., and W. A. Spencer, 1968. Cellular neurophysiological approaches in the study of learning. *Physiol. Rev.* 48:65–134.

Kandel, E. R., and L. Tauc, 1965a. Heterosynaptic facilitation in the neurons of the abdominal ganglion of *Aplysia depilans. J. Physiol.* (*Lond.*) 181:1–27.

Kandel, E. R., and L. Tauc, 1965b. Mechanism of heterosynaptic facilitation in the giant cell of the abdominal ganglion of *Aplysia depilans. J. Physiol.* (*Lond.*) 181:28–47.

Kehoe, J. S., 1969. Single presynaptic neuron mediates a two component postsynaptic inhibition. *Nature* (*Lond.*) 221:866–868.

Kehoe, J. S., 1972. Three acetylcholine receptors in *Aplysia* neurons. *J. Physiol.* (*Lond.*) 225:115–146.

Kennedy, D., A. I. Selverston, and M. P. Remler, 1969. Analysis of restricted neural networks. *Science* 164:1488–1496.

Konorski, J., 1948. *Conditioned Reflexes and Neuron Organization.* London: Cambridge University Press.

Konorski, J., 1967. *Integrative Activity of the Brain; an Inter-Disciplinary Approach.* Chicago: University of Chicago Press.

Kuba, K., 1970. Effects of catecholamines on the neuromuscular junction in the rat diaphragm. *J. Physiol.* (*Lond.*) 211:551–570.

Kupfermann, I., T. J. Carew, and E. R. Kandel, 1973. Local, reflex and central commands controlling gill and siphon movements in *Aplysia.* (In preparation.)

Kupfermann, I., V. Castellucci, H. Pinsker, and E. Kandel, 1970. Neuronal correlates of habituation and dishabituation of the gill-withdrawal reflex in *Aplysia. Science* 167:1743–1745.

Kupfermann, I., and E. R. Kandel, 1968. Reflex function of some identifiable cells in *Aplysia. Physiologist* 27:348.

Kupfermann, I., and E. R. Kandel, 1969. Neuronal controls of a behavioral response mediated by the abdominal ganglion of *Aplysia. Science* 164:847–850.

Kupfermann, I., and M. Kesselman, 1968. Withdrawal reflexes in intact and "deganglionated" *Aplysia californica.* Cited in Kandel and Spencer, 1968.

Kupfermann, I., H. Pinsker, V. Castellucci, and E. R. Kandel, 1971. Central and peripheral control of gill movements in *Aplysia. Science* 174:1252–1256.

Larrabee, M. G., and D. W. Bronk, 1947. Prolonged facilitation of synaptic excitation in sympathetic ganglia. *J. Neurophysiol.* 10:139–154.

Lasek, R. J., and W. J. Dower, 1971. *Aplysia californica*: Analysis of nuclear DNA in individual nuclei of giant neurons. *Science* 172:278–280.

Lukowiak, K., and J. W. Jacklet, 1972. Habituation and

dishabituation: Interactions between peripheral and central nervous systems in *Aplysia*. *Science* 178:1306–1308.

MACPHERSON, S. J., V. DEES, and G. C. GRINDLEY, 1949. The effect of knowledge of results on learning and performance. III. The influence of the time interval between trials. *Quart. J. Exp. Psych.* 1:167–174.

MARTIN, A. R., and G. PILAR, 1964. Presynaptic events during post-tetanic potentiation and facilitation in the airan ciliary ganglion. *J. Physiol.* 175:740–746.

MARTIN, A. R., and W. O. WICKELGREN, 1971. Sensory cells in the spinal cord of the sea lamprey. *J. Physiol.* (*Lond.*) 212: 65–83.

MAYERI, E., I. KUPFERMANN, J. KOESTER, and E. R. KANDEL, 1971. Neural coordination of heart rate and gill contraction in *Aplysia*. *Am. Zool.* 11(244):667.

MCCAMAN, R. E., and S. A. DEWHURST, 1970. Choline acetyltransferase in individual neurons of *Aplysia californica*. *J. Neurochem.* 17:1421–1426.

NEWBY, N. A., 1972. Habituation to light and spontaneous activity in the isolated siphon of *Aplysia*: The effects of synaptically active pharmacological agents. Ph.D. Thesis. Case Western Reserve University.

NICHOLLS, J. G., and D. PURVES, 1970. Monosynaptic chemical and electrical connexions between sensory and motor cells in the central nervous system of the leech. *J. Physiol.* (*Lond.*) 209:647–667.

PAVLOV, I. P., 1927. *Conditioned Reflexes*. (G. V. Anrep, trans.) London: Oxford University Press.

PEEKE, H. V. S., M. J. HERZ, and J. E. GALLAGHER, 1971. Changes in aggressive interaction in adjacently territorial convict cichlids (*Cichlasoma nigrofasciatum*): A study of habituation. *Behavior* 40:43–54.

PERETZ, B., 1969. Central neuron initiation of periodic gill movements. *Science* 166:1167–1172.

PERETZ, B., 1970. Habituation and dishabituation in the absence of a central nervous system. *Science* 169:379–381.

PINSKER, H., T. CAREW, and E. R. KANDEL, 1973. Long-term sensitization of a defensive withdrawal reflex in *Aplysia*. (In preparation.)

PINSKER, H., and E. R. KANDEL, 1967. Contingent modification of an endogenous bursting rhythm by monosynaptic inhibition. *Physiologist* 10:279.

PINSKER, H., I. KUPFERMANN, V. CASTELLUCCI, and E. KANDEL, 1970. Habituation and dishabituation of the gill-withdrawal reflex in *Aplysia*. *Science* 167:1740–1742.

RALL, T. W., and A. G. GILMAN, 1970. The role of cyclic AMP in the nervous system. *Neurosci. Res. Prog. Bull.* 8:221–323.

RASMUSSEN, H., 1970. Cell communication, calcium ion, and cyclic adenosine monophosphate. *Science* 170:404–412.

ROVAINEN, C. M., 1967. Physiological and anatomical studies on large neurons of central nervous system of the sea lamprey (*Petromyzon marinus*). I. Müller and Mauthner cells. *J. Neurophysiol.* 30:1000–1023.

SCHWARTZ, J. H., V. F. CASTELLUCCI, and E. R. KANDEL, 1971. Functioning of identified neurons and synapses in abdominal ganglion of *Aplysia* in absence of protein synthesis. *J. Neurophysiol.* 34:939–953.

SHARPLESS, S., and H. JASPER, 1956. Habituation of the arousal reaction. *Brain* 79:655–680.

SHERMAN, R. G., and H. L. ATWOOD, 1971. Synaptic facilitation: Long term neuromuscular facilitation in crustacea. *Science* 171:248–250.

SOKOLOV, E. N., 1963. *Perception and the Conditioned Reflex*. (S. W. Waydenfeld, trans.) Oxford: Pergamon Press.

SPENCER, W. A., and R. S. APRIL, 1970. Plastic properties of monosynaptic pathways in mammals. In *Short-Term Changes in Neural Activity and Behavior*, G. Horn and R. A. Hinde, eds. London: Cambridge University Press, pp. 433–474.

SPENCER, W. A., R. F. THOMPSON, and D. R. NEILSON, JR., 1966. Response decrement of the flexion reflex in the acute spinal cat and transient restoration by strong stimuli. *J. Neurophysiol.* 29:221–239.

SPERRY, R. W., 1965. Selective communication in nerve nets: Impulse specificity vs. connection specificity. *Neurosci. Res. Prog. Bull.* 3(5):37–43.

STEPHENS, C. L., 1972. Progressive decrements in the activity of *Aplysia* neurons following repeated intracellular stimulation. Ph.D. Thesis, University of California, Los Angeles.

STRUMWASSER, F., 1965. The demonstration and manipulation of a circadian rhythm in a single neuron. In *Circadian Clocks*, J. Aschoff, ed. Amsterdam: North-Holland Publishing, pp. 442–462.

STRUMWASSER, F., 1967. Types of information stored in single neurons. In *Invertebrate Nervous Systems: Their Significance for Mammalian Neurophysiology*, C. A. G. Wiersma, ed. Chicago: University of Chicago Press, pp. 291–319.

STRUMWASSER, F., 1973. This volume.

TAUC, L., 1962. Identification of active membrane areas in the giant neuron of *Aplysia*. *J. Gen. Physiol.* 45:1099–1115.

TAUC, L., 1965. Presynaptic inhibition in the abdominal ganglion of *Aplysia*. *J. Physiol.* (*Lond.*) 181:282–307.

TAUC, L., 1966. Physiology of the nervous system. In *Physiology of Mollusca*, Vol. 2, K. M. Wilbur and C. M. Yonge, eds. New York: Academic Press, pp. 387–454.

TAUC, L., 1967. Transmission in invertebrate and vertebrate ganglia. *Physiol. Rev.* 47:521–593.

TAUC, L., and H. M. GERSCHENFELD, 1961. Cholinergic transmission mechanisms for both excitation and inhibition in molluscan central synapses. *Nature* (*Lond.*) 192:366–367.

THORPE, W. H., 1963. *Learning and Instinct in Animals*, 2nd Ed. London: Methuen.

TINBERGEN, N., 1951. *The Study of Instinct*. Oxford: Clarendon Press.

WALL, P. D., 1970. Habituation and post-tetanic potentiation in the spinal cord. In *Short-Term Changes in Neural Activity and Behavior*, G. Horn and R. A. Hinde, eds. London: Cambridge University Press, pp. 181–210.

WAZIRI, R., and E. R. KANDEL, 1969. Organization of inhibition in abdominal ganglion of *Aplysia*. III. Interneurons mediating inhibition. *J. Neurophysiol.* 32:520–539.

WEISKRANTZ, L., 1970. A long-term view of short-term memory in psychology. In *Short-Term Changes in Neural Activity and Behavior*, G. Horn and R. A. Hinde, eds. London: Cambridge University Press, pp. 63–74.

WICKELGREN, B. G., 1967. Habituation of spinal interneurons. *J. Neurophysiol.* 30:1424–1438.

WILSON, D. L., 1970. Molecular weight distribution of proteins synthesized in single identified neurons of *Aplysia*. *J. Gen. Physiol.* 57:26–40.

WOODWORTH, R. S., and H. SCHLOSBERG, 1954. *Experimental Psychology*, 2nd Ed. New York: Holt, Rinehart and Winston.

ZUCKER, R. S., 1972. Crayfish escape behavior and central synapses. II. Physiological mechanisms underlying behavioral habituation. *J. Neurophysiol.* 35:621–637.

32 Characterization of Connectivity among Invertebrate Motor Neurons by Cross Correlation of Spike Trains

WILLIAM B. KRISTAN, JR.

ABSTRACT The cross-correlation histograms generated from spike trains of neuron pairs can detect connections between cells and common input to them. They can help distinguish between these modes of connectivity, even when the spikes occur in bursts. Such histograms were used to detect and quantitate the connections among and to motor neurons in invertebrate preparations. One of these is the group of motor cells involved in swimming in the leech; another is the motor fibers for slow movements of the tail in the crayfish. Electrotonic connections among motor neurons are correlated with behavior in these two systems but not to the extent shown by similar connections in motor systems with a more limited, stereotyped behavioral repertoire.

MANY INVERTEBRATE motor neurons, unlike their vertebrate counterparts, are individually distinguishable. In the leech, for example, Ann Stuart (1970) showed that the five different groups of muscles controlling the behavior of the body wall are differently innervated by identifiable motor neurons. Each segment has two homologous sets of 14 excitatory motor and 3 inhibitory neurons, one set controlling each side. No two motor neurons on each side have exactly the same properties. For instance, of the six motor neurons supplying the layer of longitudinal muscles of each half-segment of the body wall, one called the *L cell* innervates longitudinal muscle fibers in the entire half-segment; another innervates fibers only in the dorsolateral quadrant and a third only those in the ventrolateral quadrant; three others supply only dorsal, lateral, or ventral longitudinal muscle fibers. Of the two inhibitory neurons, one innervates the dorsolateral and the other the ventrolateral quadrant.

Different behavioral acts must necessarily involve different sets of these motor neurons. For instance, Nicholls and Purves (1970) have shown that the L cell is probably responsible for the symmetrical shortening reflex seen in leeches when they are touched. Tactile sensory neurons strongly excite the L cells and cause shortening of all longitudinal muscles on both sides of the segment. The symmetric shortening of the two sides of a segment is assured by a very effective electrotonic junction between the two homologous L cells in each segment (Stuart, 1970).

Swimming in the leech is the result of repeated passages of a head-to-tail wave of alternate contractions of the dorsal and ventral longitudinal muscles in successive segments. This behavior must be caused by phase-locked alternating activity in each set of motor neurons that innervate only dorsal or ventral longitudinal muscles. A study has been recently begun on the neural basis of swimming in the leech (Kristan, Stent, and Ort, unpublished). Extracellular recordings in peripheral regions of segmental nerves in swimming animals repeatedly revealed neurons that generate bursts of spikes only while either the dorsal or the ventral longitudinal muscles are contracting. Intracellular recordings identified some as motor neurons that innervate only the dorsal or ventral longitudinal muscles. To ascertain whether connections among motor neurons are responsible for the pattern of spike activity during swimming, simultaneous intracellular recordings from two neurons at a time are helpful. But, since the spike amplitude recorded from cell bodies of many of the leech motor neurons is quite small, even quite effective synaptic potentials might not be detected, and hence existing connections might be missed. Cross-correlation histograms are generated from the extracellularly recorded spike trains to overcome this problem.

Generation and interpretation of cross-correlation histograms

Cross-correlation histograms measure the likelihood that spikes in two neurons occur at particular times relative to one another (Perkel et al., 1967; Gerstein and Perkel, 1972). For example, two neurons that have excitatory synapses on one another tend to generate spikes at the same time. The strength of this tendency depends on the

WILLIAM B. KRISTAN, JR. Department of Molecular Biology, University of California, Berkeley strengths of the excitatory connections, whereas the relative timing depends upon synaptic delays and the time course of the synaptic potentials; both can be obtained from cross-correlation histograms. Common excitatory input also causes two neurons to generate spikes at nearly the same time.

Figure 1A shows data from two cells which are mutually excitatory, whereas Figure 1B shows data from two cells receiving a common excitatory input. These patterns of connections had been determined by intracellular recordings which, in these pairs of neurons, clearly show synaptic potentials (Hagiwara and Morita, 1962; Kristan, 1971).

Mutually excitatory connections

The paired *colossal* or Retzius cell bodies in each ganglion of the medicinal leech are electrotonically coupled. Nearly every spike in one cell causes a spike in the other, unless the latter is in a refractory state. This strong connection is demonstrated by their nearly superimposable spike time records as shown in Figure 1A1.

In order to generate the cross-correlation histogram between two spike trains, the intervals between each spike in one cell and every spike in the other cell are scored only during some finite time period before and after each reference spike. Positive values are given to cross-intervals in which the second cell's spikes occur later than the reference spike and negative values when the second cell's spikes occur earlier.

The resolution to which cross-intervals are measured and the length of time sampled before and after each spike depend upon the data to be analyzed. For instance, inspection of long spike train records of two Retzius cells showed that the cross-intervals were all less than 13 msec or more than 100 msec. Hence, the part of the histogram that bears on the connectivity of these two cells was the range from -13 to $+13$ msec. In this case, the time resolution of 0.5 msec best showed the time course of the excitation of each cell on the other.

As can be seen in Figure 1A2, there is little tendency for the two cells to generate spikes within 2 msec of one another. There is, however, a strong tendency for cell B spikes to occur 2 to 6.5 msec after those in cell A, and for cell A spikes to occur 3 to 12 msec after cell B spikes. These tendencies are due to the depolarizing electrotonic potentials generated in each cell by spikes in the other (Figure 1A3). These intracellular recordings show that both cells

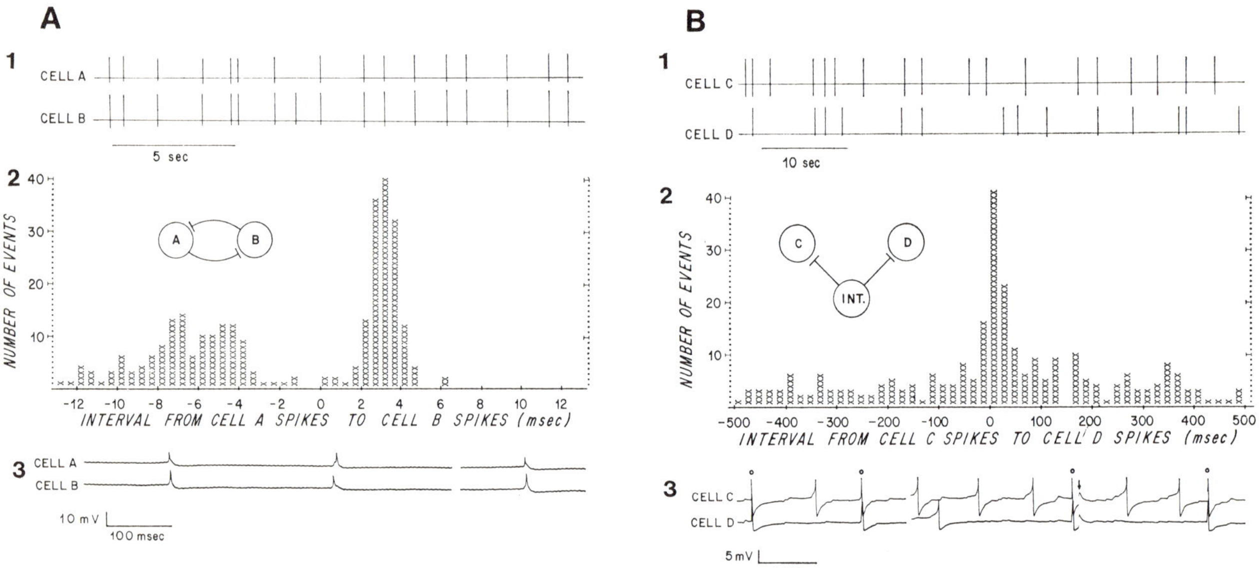

FIGURE 1 Recordings and cross-correlation histograms of the spike activity in pairs of neurons which show nearly synchronous spike times. (A1) Times of occurrence of spikes in the two Retzius cells in the same ganglion of a medicinal leech (simulation of extracellular record using data from intracellular recording). (A2) Cross-correlation histogram generated from 280 spike pairs from the same two cells. The inset shows the manner of connection between the cells, the contacts being excitatory electrical synapses. Bin width = 0.5 msec. (A3) Intracellular recordings of the same two cells, showing the activity caused in one cell by an action potential in the other. (B1) Spike occurrence times from recordings of two cells C and D, in the right pleural ganglion of *Aplysia*. (B2) Cross-correlation histogram using 252 spikes in cell C and 234 spikes in cell D. Inset shows the cause of the peak in the histogram, a common interneuron which provides strong excitatory input to both cells. Bin width = 20 msec. (B3) Intracellular recordings from cells C and D. The arrow marks input from the common interneuron, which causes spikes in both cells on the occurrences marked with dots.

had a progressive, spontaneous depolarization of their membrane potential. In the present data, this slow depolarization caused 148 spikes in cell A (exemplified by the first and third spikes in the upper record in Figure 1A3) and 216 spikes in cell B (exemplified by the second spike in the lower record in Figure 1A3). These spontaneously generated spikes caused concurrent depolarizations in the other cell, which were usually sufficient to cause it to fire. The spikes in the follower cell also generated depolarizations in the leader cell that never caused spikes because of refractoriness in the leader cell. In the 148 cases in which cell A fired first, the resulting depolarization always caused a spike in cell B, usually on the early part of the rising phase of the depolarization. When cell B fired first (216 times), the resulting depolarization was less effective, causing cell A spikes in only 132 cases, which usually occurred near the peak of the excitatory potential. This asymmetry in synaptic effectiveness is reflected in the cross-correlation histogram shown in Figure 1A2. There are 148 points in the positive-valued peak and 132 points in the negative-valued peak. In addition, the negative-valued peak has a longer delay and is more dispersed than the positive-valued peak.

These data were selected to show the appearance of excitatory potentials of different effectiveness in a cross-correlation histogram. The more usual finding is that the more posterior Retzius cell (B) always reaches threshold first and is, therefore, generally the leader cell (Lent, 1972). In such cases, there would be only a negative-valued peak in the cross-correlation histogram. The asymmetry in synaptic effectiveness may be due to the fact that the more anterior Retzius cell (A) in each ganglion has a longer proximal axon (Charles Lent, personal communication). Spike potentials generated by the posterior cell (B) might, therefore, be more attenuated because they are entering a larger cell volume than similar potentials passing in the other direction.

Common excitatory input

Many neurons in the pleural ganglia of the sea hare *Aplysia* show simultaneously occurring large synaptic potentials (EPSPs) believed to result from spikes in a single presynaptic interneuron (Kristan, 1971). EPSPs in two such cells are shown in Figure 1B3. Both cells usually generated spikes (dots), but not always (arrow), when this potential appeared. The postsynaptic cells are not interconnected nor do they receive any other major common input. These cells do generate spikes not caused by the common input, however, and thus show a lesser tendency to fire at the same time (Figure 1B1) than do electrotonically coupled cells (Figure 1A1).

The cross-correlation histogram (Figure 1B2) shows that the long duration of the common excitatory potential produces a broad peak. If the common excitatory potential arrived simultaneously at both cells and was equally effective, the peak would be centered at zero. The peak is centered at 17 msec to the right because the common input, whose arrival time at each cell of the pair varied by less than 1 msec in intracellular records, was more effective in cell C than in cell D.

A peak produced by common input is distinguishable from one produced by synaptic excitation between two cells because it includes very short cross-intervals, e.g. 0.5 msec, or less.

Not every point in the central peak resulted from the common input, because some spikes were due to unrelated excitation of the two cells. The cross-correlation histogram cannot be used to tell *which* of the near-synchronous spikes were chance occurrences, but it can be used to tell *how many* there were. Since all unrelated spikes in the two cells will occur at all cross-intervals with equal likelihood, the cross-correlation, when extended to times that are long relative to the known duration of the input, will provide this number per time unit.

The number due to common input is therefore the total number of points in the peak less the number due to chance. In Figure 1B2, the average number of points per column beyond 200 msec is 3.23. This means that of the 175 spikes generated in cell D within 200 msec of cell C spikes, 65 were due to unrelated excitation and 110 to the common input. The number of mutual spikes caused by the common input, based on counts from the intracellular records, was 104, thus checking well with that of the cross-correlation histogram. Common input which causes a spike in only one or neither cell is not detected by the cross-correlation histogram. Therefore, without intracellular recordings, the 110 common input spikes might be assigned to either 110 common excitatory potentials that were 100% effective or to many more individually less effective ones, or a mixture of the two. When two cells have all their input in common, but all EPSPs are small, the chances of any particular presynaptic impulse bringing both cells simultaneously to threshold would be small, and the cross-correlation histogram would show no peak at zero. Consequently, the size of peaks in the cross-correlation histogram indicates only the lower limit of the number of common excitatory potentials.

Synergistic leech motor neurons

During swimming, synergistic leech motor neurons generate bursts of spikes at one phase of the swim cycle and are silent between bursts. In different cells the bursts differ in duration but overlap in time. Such bursts probably result primarily from periodic bursts in presynaptic fibers common to all synergistic motor neurons (see the discussion section).

Figure 2a shows extracellular recordings from three peripheral nerves on the same side of one segment in a swimming leech. Spikes from only one neuron appear in the nerve A recording, while both the nerve B and C recordings show many classes, each from a single neuron, of spikes distinguishable by their size and shape. The spikes in nerve A are from a motor neuron, cell A, that fires during contraction of the dorsal longitudinal muscles (Lent, unpublished). The largest negative-going spikes in nerve B and the largest spikes in C are also from motor neurons (cells B and C) that generate bursts at the same time.

The shape of the broad peak in the cross-correlation histogram of two of these cells depends upon the pattern of spikes within the burst in each cell. If each neuron generated spikes at a nearly constant but different frequency, the peak would be binomial in appearance. The spike frequency in leech motor neuron bursts is nearly constant at the beginning of the burst but decreases sharply at the end. This gives long tails to the peaks, making them appear more normally distributed.

Burst duration varied from 50 to more than 500 msec in the three cells, and relative onset times of the bursts also varied somewhat. However, the means of the broad peaks in their cross-correlation histograms, shown in Figures 2b to 2d (data from different preparations), are each within 15 msec of zero. Therefore, the center of the bursts in all three cells is consistently at nearly the same time.

As is demonstrated in Figure 1, large common excitatory potentials or interconnections will cause one or more peaks at or near zero that are no wider than the duration of the individual synaptic potentials. The central area of the cross-correlation histogram of cells A and C (Figure 2b) does not show any significant narrow peaks. Therefore, these cells probably have neither an excitatory interconnection nor a common source of large excitatory potentials. However, in the cross-correlation histogram of B and C, a narrow peak occurs in the -5 to 10 msec cross-interval range. Since this peak crosses zero, cells B and C probably receive large excitatory potentials from a common source. The 84 points in this peak represent the minimum number of the 695 spikes in B and 1432 spikes in C that were caused by this common input.

The cross-correlation histogram of cells A and B (Figure 2d) has a narrow peak at $+5$ to $+10$ msec, implying an excitatory input from A to B. The 52 points mean that 6.5% of the activity in cell B resulted from this input by cell A.

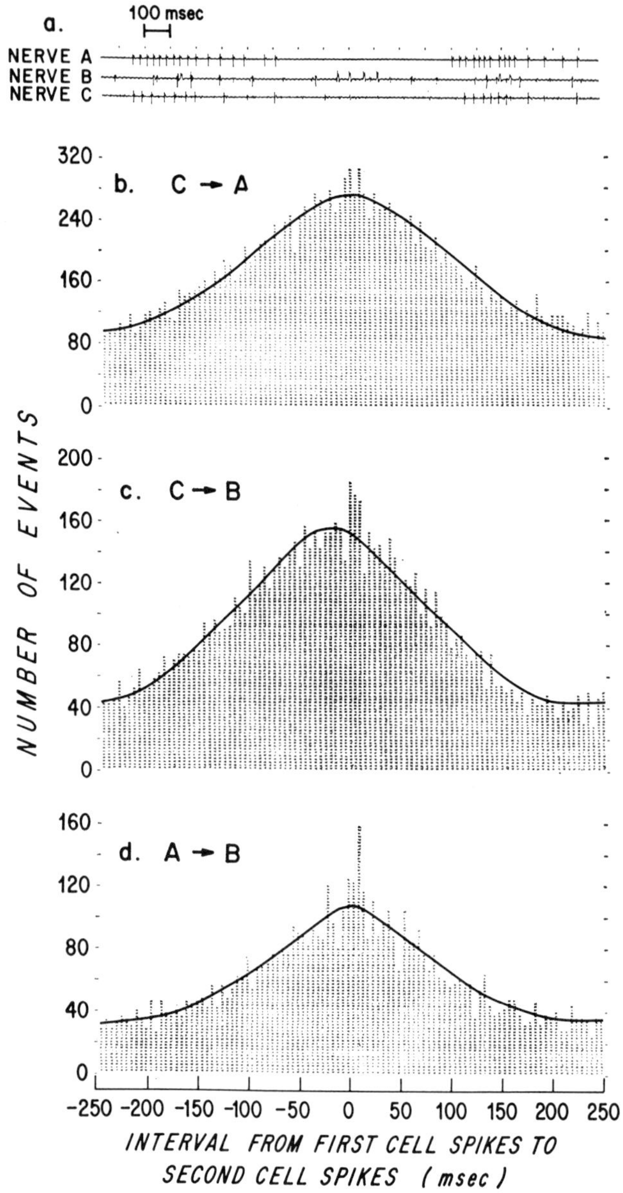

FIGURE 2 Connections among three synergistic leech motor neurons. (a) Extracellular recordings showing three motor neurons that generate bursts of spikes during dorsal longitudinal muscle contraction. Spikes in the nerve A recording are from a single cell called "A," the most negative-going spikes in the nerve B recording are from the cell called "B," and the largest spikes in the nerve C recording are from the cell called "C." (b) Cross-correlation histogram of 1990 A spikes and 2187 C spikes. For this histogram and that of Figures 2c, 2d, and 4c, the solid line enveloping the broad peak was determined by drawing a symmetric bell-shaped curve on the histogram. The actual value in each column was then subtracted from the value predicted by the curve. The whole curve was then shifted up or down by the amount necessary to make the sum of these differences zero. (c) Cross-correlation histogram of 695 B spikes and 1432 C spikes. (d) Cross-correlation histogram of 1125 A spikes and 803 B spikes. Each column in all histograms represents 5 msec.

Synergistic crayfish motor neurons

Figure 3 shows data of William Tatton which were obtained by extracellular recordings from motor neurons which control posture and slow movements of the crayfish tail. The anatomy of this motor system is similar in many respects to the leech longitudinal muscle system. Each of the first five segments in the crayfish tail has a dorsal and a ventral longitudinal set of slow muscles. Contraction in the dorsal muscles causes a lifting or extension of the tail, whereas ventral muscle contraction causes dropping or flexion of the tail. There are six neurons innervating each flexor and extensor muscle on one side of one segment, five being excitatory, with different areas of innervation, and one being inhibitory (Kennedy and Takeda, 1965).

Figure 3a is a recording in which spikes from one group of six flexor neurons can be seen. Typical spikes from the two largest excitatory neurons are marked. Cell 6 fires in bursts of 2 to 4 spikes. Cell 4 is more tonically active, but increases its frequency during cell 6 bursts.

Figure 3b shows a cross-correlation histogram of spike activity in cells 6 and 4 while random electrical shocks were delivered to a sensory nerve. The 0 to +20 msec cross-interval column constitutes a highly significant narrow peak containing 165 points. When a 1 msec time resolution was used, the peak was restricted to the +3 to +5 msec columns, suggesting an excitatory connection from cell 6 to cell 4. Cell 6 generated 368 spikes and 165 of them caused spikes in cell 4.

The solid horizontal line in the histogram marks the average number of events per column at long cross-interval times. There is a broad peak above this line, implying that there are cell 4 bursts that overlap with those of cell 6. The total width of this peak is about 1300 msec. Since cell 6 bursts last no longer than 100 msec, the cell 4 bursts must be considerably longer and are, therefore, only partially due to the excitation from cell 6.

Bilateral homologous leech motor neurons

When a few middle segments of a leech are opened and prevented by fixation from contracting, the free front and

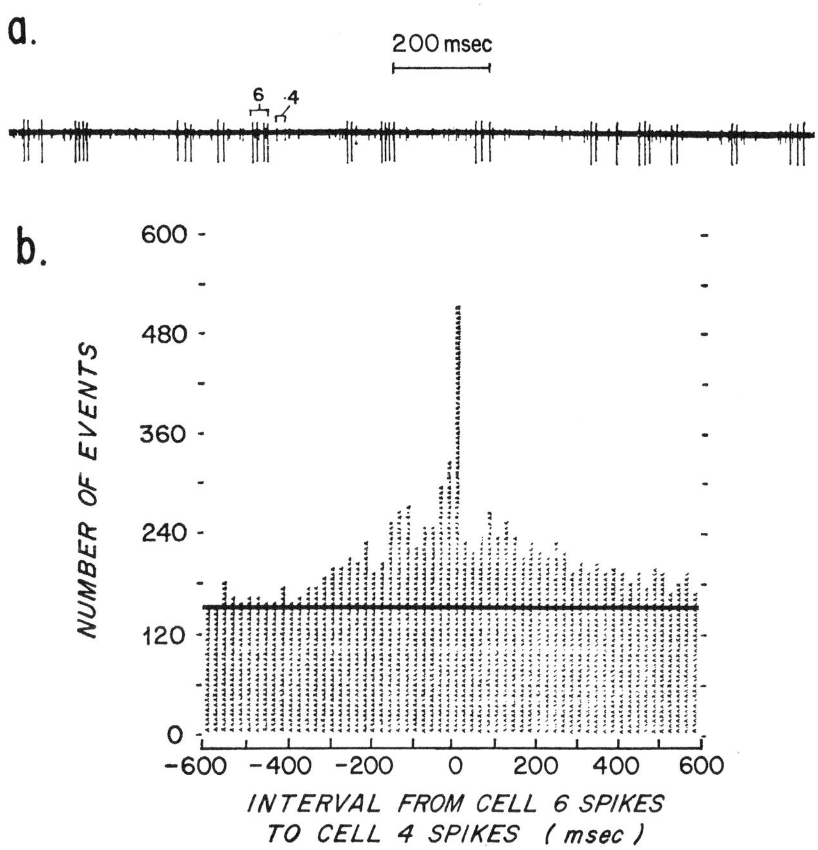

FIGURE 3 Connections between two crayfish tail motor neurons. (a) Extracellular recordings from a peripheral nerve to the flexor muscles showing spikes in all six motor neurons. Typical spikes from the two largest excitatory flexor motor neurons have been labeled "6" and "4," according to the convention of Kennedy and Takeda, 1965. (b) Cross-correlation histogram of 368 cell 6 spikes and 4810 cell 4 spikes. Each column represents 20 msec. (Courtesy of W. Tatton.)

back parts of the animal can still swim in unison. Under these conditions homologous motor neurons on the two sides of a single segment generate very similar bursts of spikes during swimming episodes, as shown in Figure 4a.

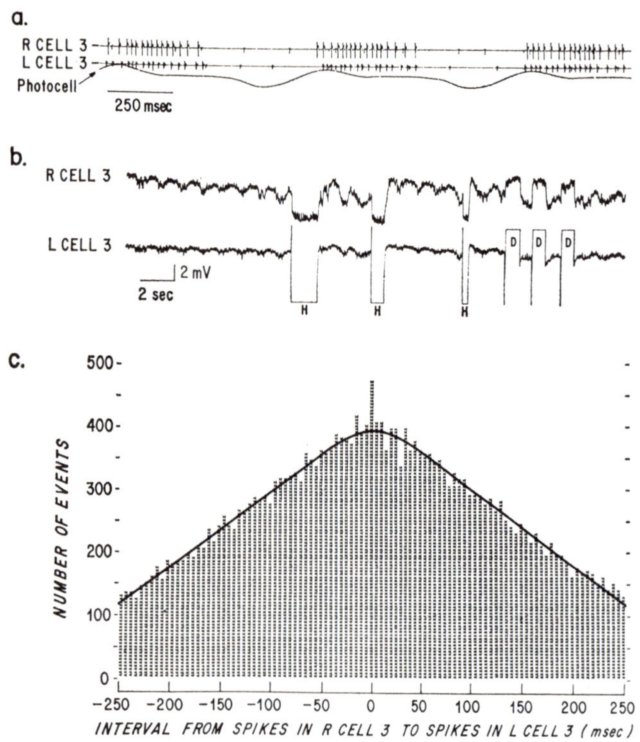

FIGURE 4 Functional strength of an electrotonic junction between bilaterally symmetric motor neurons. (a) Extracellular recordings from homologous peripheral nerves on opposite sides of the same segment in a swimming leech. The largest spikes in each recording are from bilaterally symmetric motor neurons called "cell 3." The bottom trace shows variations in the voltage from a photocell that indicate swimming movements in the anterior part of the leech. (b) Intracellular recordings from the cell bodies of the same two cells in another preparation. Hyperpolarizing (H) and depolarizing (D) currents were passed through the recording electrode into the left cell 3. Since both polarities of current pulses produce corresponding membrane potential changes in the right cell 3, the two cells are electrotonically coupled. (c) Cross-correlation of 2659 spikes in the right cell 3 and 2549 spikes in the left cell 3. Each column represents 5 msec.

The largest spikes in each extracellular record are from two bilaterally homologous motor neurons in a midbody ganglion, whose somata positions within the ganglion are known. Their names, "cell 3," derive from an arbitrary numbering of the motor cells (Kristan, Stent and Ort, unpublished). Intracellular recordings from the two cell bodies show that they are electrotonically coupled (Figure 4b). Both hyperpolarizing and depolarizing potentials induced by passing current into the left cell spread to the right one. Therefore, those two cells are connected in the same manner as the Retzius cells.

If this interconnection were as effective for mutual excitation as in the Retzius cells, the similarity of the bursts in the two cells would be explained. Intracellular recordings were of little use in determining the effectiveness, because in the cell bodies there is little or, as in Figure 4b, no evidence of the spikes recordable in the peripheral nerves.

A cross-correlation histogram was generated from extracellular recordings to measure the effectiveness of spikes in each cell on spike generation in the other. The data from 280 bursts were used to reduce variability in the height of columns in the histogram so that a narrow peak at zero time would be detectable. Such a narrow peak of 5 msec duration was found but contained only 65 points, whereas over 5200 spikes were generated in the two cells. Thus only 1.3% of them could be attributed to excitation passing across the electrotonic junction, showing that in this instance mutual excitation by an electrotonic junction is only of very minor functional importance and that common synaptic input must be the reason for the concurrent bursts.

Discussion

Neither intracellular recording nor cross-histogram analysis can, under all circumstances, unambiguously describe the relationships between individual cells. For instance on the basis of Figure 2, cell A is thought to excite cell B whereas B and C are thought to receive effective common excitation. These conclusions derive from comparing the timing of the narrow peaks in their cross-correlation histograms with those in Figure 1, which were obtained from cells of known connectivity. Unfortunately, alternate interpretations are easily imagined for either type of histogram. The single peak in positive time in Figure 2d might result from common excitation which takes longer to reach cell B. The wider peak in Figure 2c might result from a combination of excitation and an excitatory synapse from cell C to B, with the separate peaks merging into a single one which crosses zero cross-interval time.

Efforts have been made to distinguish between such possibilities on the basis of further analysis of the same spike trains (Gerstein, 1970; Moore et al., 1970). Another technique is possible if the neurons can be individually stimulated. If the frequency of spikes were increased solely in cell A and if it were presynaptic to cell B, the amplitude of the peak in their cross-correlation histogram would be increased. If the peak is due to common input, it would remain the same size. Likewise, activation of cell B or C by themselves should not change the amplitude of their cross-correlation peak if they receive only common input and are not interconnected.

The connections among motor neurons responsible for swimming in the leech are weaker than those found among other motor neuron systems in invertebrates (see Selverston later in this part). Strong synaptic connections among motor neurons severely limit their behavioral repertoire. For instance, the strong excitation of cell 6 on cell 4 in crayfish abdominal system makes it impossible to activate cell 6 without increasing activity in cell 4. In fact, both cells cause contraction in the same muscle, with cell 6 typically being active only during strong contractions (Kennedy and Takeda, 1965). The synaptic contact between them increases the amount of excitation that cell 6 spikes deliver to the muscle. Similarly the very effective electrotonic junction between L cell of the leech (Stuart, 1970) that insures symmetric shortening of a segment does so at the expense of being able to use these motor neurons in turning.

The same muscles the leech uses to swim are used in different combinations to walk, turn, and maintain an upright position in swimming. Therefore, these motor neurons must be less fettered by interconnections, and most of the excitation generating bursts in leech motor neurons, therefore, must come from common input. However, the amount of common input due to individually effective synaptic excitations is small, as shown in Figure 2. Presumably, the common excitation results from summed potentials that are individually weak. Alternately, the motor neurons could receive their excitation from a common presynaptic cell that generates only slow oscillations of its membrane potential but no spikes (Mendelson, 1971).

ACKNOWLEDGMENTS I would like to thank William Tatton and Charles Lent for the use of unpublished data and Donald Perkel for assistance in using his spike train analysis programs. I am also grateful to Donald Kennedy, C. A. G. Wiersma, Theodore Bullock, and especially to Gunther Stent for suggestions in the preparation of this manuscript. This work was done at both Stanford University and the University of California at Berkeley. It was supported by National Science Foundation Research Grant GB 31933X, and a National Science Foundation Postdoctoral Fellowship.

REFERENCES

GERSTEIN, G. L., 1970. Functional association of neurons: Detection and interpretation. In *The Neurosciences Second Study Program*, F. O. Schmitt, ed. New York: Rockefeller University Press, pp. 648–660.

GERSTEIN, G. L., and D. H. PERKEL, 1972. Mutual temporal relationships among neuronal spike trains. *Biophys. J.* 12: 453–473.

HAGIWARA, S., and H. MORITA, 1962. Electrotonic transmission between two nerve cells in leech ganglion. *J. Neurophysiol.* 25:721–731.

KENNEDY, D., and K. TAKEDA, 1965. Reflex control of abdominal flexor muscles in the crayfish. II. The tonic system. *J. Exp. Biol.* 43:229–246.

KRISTAN, W. B., JR., 1971. Plasticity of firing patterns in neurons of *Aplysia* pleural ganglion. *J. Neurophysiol.* 34:321–336.

LENT, C. M., 1972. Electrophysiology of Retzius cells of segmental ganglia in the horse leech, *Haemopus marmorata* (Say). *Comp. Biochem. Physiol.* 42A:857–862.

MENDELSON, M., 1971. Oscillator neuron in crustacean ganglia. *Science* 171:1170–1173.

MOORE, G. P., J. P. SEGUNDO, D. H. PERKEL, and H. LEVITAN, 1970. Statistical signs of synaptic interaction in neurons. *Biophys. J.* 9:876–900.

NICHOLLS, J. G., and D. PURVES, 1970. Monosynaptic chemical and electrical connections between sensory and motor cells in the central nervous system of the leech. *J. Physiol.* 209:647–667.

PERKEL, D. H., G. L. GERSTEIN, and G. P. MOORE, 1967. Neuronal spike trains and stochastic point processes. II. Simultaneous spike trains. *Biophys. J.* 7:419–440.

STUART, A. E., 1970. Physiological and morphological properties of motoneurons in the central nervous system of the leech. *J. Physiol.* 209:627–646.

33 Connections among Neurons of Different Types in Crustacean Nervous Systems

DONALD KENNEDY

ABSTRACT Crustacean nervous systems share many of the advantages found in other invertebrate preparations: Large cell size, restricted numbers of neurons, and consistent neurogeography. In addition, their motor systems are unusually well charted and accessible, and as a result control neurons have been identified not only in terms of their connection with the sensory periphery but also in terms of the coordinated motor outputs they release. These *command fibers* appear, like the sensory interneurons, to be unique entities, each with a set of connections appropriate to an element of behavior. The identification of elements has proceeded to a point at which we are able to describe identified connections at five levels in the nervous system that are responsible for a behavioral act. Sensory neurons differ, however, from the constant, connection-specific central elements: They are added constantly during life, degenerate relatively rapidly following axonotomy, and make less rigidly specified connections with other cells. The central neurons must adjust continually to the presence of new input from this source. The fact that a relatively greater proportion of axons in the central nervous system of the adult comes from this second cell population indicates that earlier estimates of the number of interneurons and motor neurons are too high.

ALMOST EXACTLY twenty years ago, the chairman of our study team delivered a paper, *Neurons of Arthropods*, at the Cold Spring Harbor Symposium (Wiersma, 1952). Both the symposium and Dr. Wiersma's contribution proved to be bench marks in early postwar neurophysiology. The new techniques of intracellular recording were for the first time being applied to the mammalian spinal cord, and it can properly be said that our inventory of the integrative capacity of central neurons was just beginning. Wiersma was able to outline a number of respects in which the study of arthropod nerve cells might help to advance that goal. First, he pointed out that arthropods have a markedly reduced number of neurons compared with that found in vertebrates and suggested that single cells in arthropods may therefore have to perform a more complex set of integrative functions. He reviewed evidence that the lateral giant fibers of decapod Crustacea, for example, frequently conduct in both directions as a consequence of their anatomical organization, and he pointed to the broad variety of synaptic contacts made by these identified cells. Finally, he showed that the diversity of output junctions made by a single neuron can make it the trigger for a complex, highly differentiated behavioral output.

DONALD KENNEDY Department of Biological Sciences, Stanford University, Stanford, California

Since we have come to expect a good deal of Wiersma's crystal ball, it is perhaps not surprising that his remarks in 1952 provide such a useful outline for a treatment of the arthropod central nervous system in 1972. The major conceptual advances that have been made in the intervening two decades can, I think, be summarized as follows: (1) The concept of *identified cells* has been extended from its application to a few, highly specialized large neurons—the giant fibers and a few others—to embrace, if not the entire central nervous system, at least a reasonably large proportion of the central interneurons. Based mainly on studies in decapod Crustacea, it seems clear that each central interneuron in the arthropod nervous system is a unique entity, connecting with some special set of input fibers and having an equally specific array of output connections. (2) It is now widely believed that this specificity of connections in the arthropod nervous system is established in part by stereotyped branching by the neurons during development. This conclusion has been reached through the application of new dye-injection techniques that allow the spread of a fluorescent or electron-dense label throughout the processes of the cell and permit a complete reconstruction. Other neurogeographic studies in arthropods, annelids, and molluscs have shown that the arrangement of identified cell somata with respect to one another is also highly constant, as shown in the communications by Kandel, Hoyle, and Selverston elsewhere in this part. (3) Synaptic organization in arthropod neuropil, though it differs in some morphological respects from that in the vertebrate central nervous system, builds upon the same synaptic mechanisms found in vertebrates. Presynaptic inhibition, electrotonic junctions, conventional chemical EPSPs and IPSPs all occur—although in different proportions and sometimes in unexpected functional roles. (4) Many of the "complex" features of patterned motor output—reciprocity, phase-constancy, and the like—are the products not of continuous reflex control from the periphery during the execution of the behavior, but, instead, of central connections among a relatively small population of neural elements.

It is in connection with this last issue that arthropod nervous systems have seen their hardest experimental service. My late colleague, Don Wilson, reviewed this problem at the last Boulder conference (Wilson, 1970), and I therefore intend to pay relatively little attention to the important subject of pattern-generating networks. It does seem appropriate, however, to summarize the evidence for the other generalities that have emerged during the past twenty years, and then to deal with some challenges to them. I intend to focus on crustacean nervous systems entirely, for these have been a kind of "proving ground" for new technologies and insights that could then be applied to insects. In the long run, one must concede that the insects are the most promising of the organisms with "reduced" nervous systems, both because they possess a wider range of behaviors and—most important—because they have accessible genetics. Crustaceans, however, although they don't fly, sing, or reproduce well in the laboratory, do one thing better than insects: They grow. Because of their size, one can do things with them that one would hardly dream of trying on an insect unless emboldened by success with a similar but easier preparation. Thus the major technical breakthroughs in understanding neuropil—intracellular recording and dye injection—have both been first accomplished in Crustacea and then successfully exported to insects.

Identified cells

Although it was known by 1950 that a variety of animals possessed fixed numbers of unusually large, highly specialized neurons that could be identified in one preparation after another, it was not established even for the smallest divisions of these nervous systems that they consisted of arrays of "unique" cells. In his 1952 Cold Spring Harbor paper, Wiersma alluded to the stimulation of several different central neurons that evoked distinctive behavioral effects, and over the next ten years he produced a series of papers demonstrating for a much larger number of cells that there were also unique input connections. First in the circumesophageal connectives (Wiersma, 1958) then in the abdominal nervous system (Wiersma and Hughes, 1961; Wiersma and Bush, 1963), it was shown that nerve fibers with identical peripheral receptive fields could repeatedly be isolated from a particular part of the cross section of a central connective. Each such entity is unique: For example, of the set of interneurons receiving input from abdominal tactile hairs, one may connect with hairs on both sides of all six segments, another from a particular dorsal patch on only one segment, another from three, another from five, and so on; a particular locus in the periphery is multiply represented centrally, but each time it converges with a unique combination of other peripheral loci. Although the position of identified interneurons in the central connectives is not exactly constant, there is little difficulty in identifying the large ones, and the precision with which their receptive fields are repeated from animal to animal is a fact we can fully confirm. A total of about 120 interneurons (in addition to some sensory fibers) have been identified and mapped by this technique.

For the same purpose, central elements can be tested by stimulating them and seeing what happens. Wiersma first showed that stimulating fine filaments of nerve from central connectives could produce complex, stereotyped behavioral output; Wiersma and Ikeda (1964) described several such neurons that control the swimmeret rhythm and called them *command* fibers. Since then it has been shown (Kennedy et al., 1967) that impulse activity restricted to a single cell can produce coordinated motor output involving some 300 motor neurons.

In our laboratory we have attempted to establish the functional uniqueness of the premotor elements that produce the same general class of behavioral result. I will cite four systems of increasing complexity in which command interneurons can be differentiated by the details of their peripheral effect. (1) In slow abdominal flexor muscles of the crayfish, stimulation of a single central neuron produces excitation of the motor neuron, central inhibition of the motor neuron to the antagonistic muscle, and reciprocal effects on the peripheral inhibitory axons that also innervate these muscles. If one records independently from several segments, it is clear that each one produces a special segmental ratio of effect and thus encodes a particular geometry of movement (Evoy and Kennedy, 1967). (2) Extensor command fibers may excite motorneurons that go exclusively to "working" extensor muscles, or they may excite motorneurons that also innervate the receptor muscle of the muscle receptor organ. Like the activity of gamma motorneurons, this engages a myotatic reflex loop that provides for load compensation by supplying additional excitation to the extensor muscles (Fields, 1966; Fields, Evoy, and Kennedy, 1967). Thus two different command routes exist, one the equivalent of alpha activation, the other the equivalent of alpha-gamma coactivation; both are preprogrammed, and the differentiation between them is on the basis of output connections from the command interneurons. (3) In the motor systems that control positioning of an appendage in three dimensions, single command interneurons may affect output to several antagonistic sets of muscles. Command fibers produce different positions by evoking different ratios of activity in the several sets (Larimer and Kennedy, 1969). (4) Finally, interneurons commanding complex, cyclical locomotor programs in a series of appendages may produce special effects on such different parameters of the output as ratios of the alternating flexor and extensor discharges, specific portions of the dynamic range, and so on (Davis and Kennedy, 1972). For present purposes, the interesting outcome is that each central element is again unique; that is, it makes a set of connections not quite like any other interneuron and thus produces a special output pattern. Interneuronal organization on the motor side thus mirrors that on the sensory side: The cells are connected with great specificity to their output elements, and no one is just like any other.

Constancy of form

In the Cold Spring Harbor paper mentioned earlier, Wiersma described arthropod neuropil as "a complicated felt-work of nerve fibers, in which it is not possible to trace the connections." This situation was very difficult to deal with until the development of dyes that, after injection into single cells, could be expected to stay inside them and diffuse to the tips of even their finer processes. Stretton and Kravitz (1968) found that the fluorescent dye, Procion yellow, fulfilled both of these criteria and also survived subsequent fixation. They used it to reconstruct the branching pattern of a flexor inhibitor neuron in the lobster. We applied it to a series of flexor motor neurons and interneurons in the crayfish in order to test proposals about their uniqueness and the constancy of their branching and connection patterns (Remler, Selverston, and Kennedy, 1968; Kennedy, Selverston, and Remler, 1969; Selverston and Kennedy, 1969; Selverston and Remler, 1972). At least to the level of major branches, the patterns proved quite consistent for individual motor neurons, and it moreover proved possible to visualize direct connections between the fast flexor motor neurons and the central giant fibers: Connections could be physiologically verified when branches from the motor neurons appeared to contact the axis cylinders of the giant fibers and were found to be absent when such contacts were not apparent. The question of constancy in such cells is dealt with in more depth by Selverston elsewhere in this part.

Nature of the connections

The first intracellular recordings in arthropod neuropil (Preston and Kennedy, 1960; Kennedy and Preston, 1960) demonstrated all the graded forms of inhibitory and excitatory transmission that one had come to expect from central nervous structures elsewhere. Although some cell bodies of motor neurons show passive invasion by spikes (Takeda and Kennedy, 1964), most are electrically inexcitable. It is now clear that most of the interneuron somata, like the lateral giant cell illustrated in Figure 1, are so far from the sites of electrical activity in the neuropil that they are quite useless for monitoring; thus a method that has worked so well in molluscan ganglia—that of using the neurogeography of somata as the basis for a physiological identification of cells—has failed for most crustacean cells except the large motor neurons.

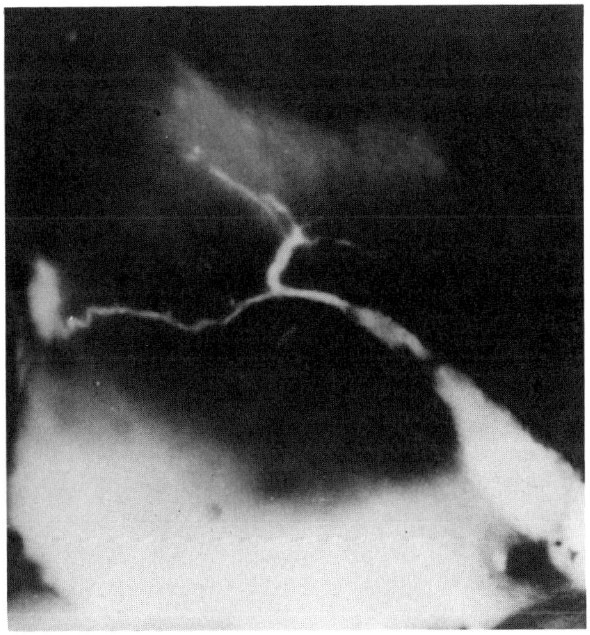

FIGURE 1 The lateral giant neuron in the third abdominal ganglion of the crayfish, injected with Procion yellow and photographed in a whole mount by fluorescence microscopy (Remler, Selverston, and Kennedy, 1968).

More recently, two more novel features of connections in neuropil have emerged. First, it is clear that dendritic branches of motor neurons and interneurons are capable of supporting all-or-none activity, and that such branch spikes summate with graded postsynaptic potentials to determine firing (Takeda and Kennedy, 1964, 1965; Sandeman, 1969). Second, a large proportion of the synaptic activity generated in sensory neuropil by afferent stimulation, or by activity in identified interneurons, is mediated by electrical connections (Zucker et al., 1971).

At this point, the correlations between structure and function in neuropil begin to break down. Although on physiological grounds many identified neurons in the crayfish central nervous system must receive electrical connections, it has not yet been possible to reveal appropriate morphological substrates for them by electron microscopy. Although "gap junctions" appear at such known sites of electrical transmission as the septum between lateral giant fibers and the junctions between giant and motor giant axons, they have not been found on the lateral giant axons in neuropil, even though electrical transmission is known to occur there (Krasne and Stirling, 1972; our own observations). Neither do they appear at other known sites of electrical transmission (Sandeman and Mendum, 1971). There are other difficulties: Even in some of the situations where electrical transmission is known to occur, synaptic vesicles are selectively concentrated at the presynaptic side of the junction. Methods of separating electrical from chemical synaptic action that are considered reliable in other situations fail to make the discrimination here: Lowered calcium and increased magnesium *do not* interfere with chemical synaptic transmission in crustacean neuropil, and conversely lowered calcium *does* affect electrotonic junctions (Asada and Bennett, 1971).

These features may perhaps best be described in connection with a specific piece of behavior; the account is taken from the work of Zucker et al. (1971). When the abdomen of a rested crayfish is tapped, the animal responds with a tail flip, incomplete in the most caudal segments, that propels it up and away from the stimulus. This behavior is known to result from a single impulse in the lateral giant fibers (Wine and Krasne, 1972), which make different connections upon motor neurons than do the medial giant fibers and produce a distinctive response (Larimer et al., 1971). It has been possible to analyze identified neurons at half a dozen hierarchial levels concerned with this behavior (Figure 2), and I treat each of them here briefly.

1. *Hair receptors* associated with the exoskeleton are deformed by the stimulus and carry impulses centrally; these have a central action at two levels. They provide an excitation to lower-order interneurons that is essentially chemical in nature, probably mediated by acetycholine (Barker et al., 1972); this response "follows the stimulus" only at relatively low frequencies. The same set of sensory neurons also makes electrical contact with higher-order interneurons, including identified cells each of which receive input in a number of adjacent body segments.

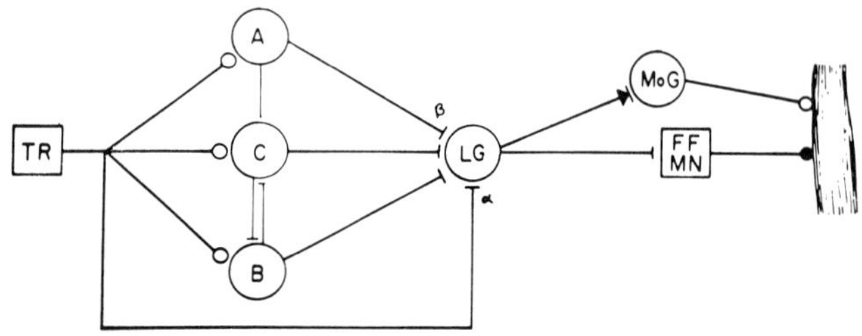

FIGURE 2 Circuit for excitation of the "tail flip" reflex by tactile stimuli. TR: tactile receptors; A: primary interneuron; B and C: second order interneurons; LG: lateral giant neuron; FFMN: fast flexor motor neuron; MoG: motor giant neuron. Circles signify chemical synapses, which show rapid depression in all cases where the circles are open; bars signify electrical synapses. (From Zucker, Kennedy, and Selverston, 1971.)

2. *Primary interneurons* receive exclusively chemical excitation from the afferents. They in turn synapse electrically on all interneurons of higher order.

3. *Multisegmental interneurons.* These receive electrical connections from primary afferents and from at least some primary interneurons and activate the lateral giant neuron electrically.

4. *Lateral giant interneuron.* This "motor" interneuron receives an exclusively electrical input from all the above elements.

5. *Motor neurons.* These are excited by the lateral giant fibers, and probably by other elements of lower order. The majority of their input is electrical. They supply chemical excitation to phasic flexor muscles of the abdomen. At the neuromuscular junctions, additional temporal labilities are introduced (Bruner and Kennedy, 1970).

This brief account emphasizes several features of the neural network involved in escape behavior. First, it is a kind of cascade, with short loops featuring electrical excitation and longer ones that are begun by a chemical stage. This last feature makes them subject to depression in response to repetition of the stimulus, and for that reason this part of the circuit shows substantial lability. The electrical component of the primary afferent volley is, by itself, unable to activate the final common neuron that acts as the behavioral trigger. Sensory neurons have a dual synaptic action, electrically exciting some neurons and chemically exciting others; both roles may be played by branches of the same sensory neuron. Finally, temporal lability is evident only at the first and last stages of the circuit.

Unfortunately, however, the only explicit statements we can make about cell identity and connectivity in this circuit involve the centrally located interneurons and motor neurons. What about the specificity of relations between this center and the sensory periphery?

Sensory neurons

Afferent axons in the arthropods develop from peripherally located cell bodies, which arise by the division and differentiation of epithelial cells. We have found that these cells differ from central neurons in their specificity of connection, in their response to axonotomy, and in their pattern of growth and development. While these new findings threaten one or two generalities about connectivity in these nervous systems, they save us from at least one potential embarrassment.

The first-stage interneuron described above, which responds to water-borne vibrations that activate exoskeletal hairs on the tail fan, has provided an opportunity to analyze the connections made by sensory fibers. A map of the peripheral region that supplies axons to the sixth ganglion via the fourth root is shown in Figure 3. Each hair sends one and sometimes two axons to the central nervous system, and these may either stop in the ganglion of entry or continue to higher levels. Hairs in the more rostral portion of the field (especially P_1, P_2, P_3, L_1 and S_1 in the figure) show higher thresholds and give more phasic responses. In experiments begun in collaboration with Allen Selverston, we have measured the conduction velocity of afferent fibers from single hairs to determine their relative size and recorded the unitary excitatory postsynaptic potentials they produced in the interneuron (Figure 4). The four or five largest proximal cells are very likely to make connections with the interneuron; they do so in at least 80 or 90% of the cases. More distally, predictions are less easy to make; cells in the central region may show a hit-or-miss pattern of connection, and in the most distal or lateral areas only an occasional hair will produce a unitary synaptic potential. There is *no* correlation between fiber diameter and synaptic efficacy, but the larger afferents are more likely to make connections.

For present purposes, the interesting feature is that the neurons belonging to this system do not show the rigorously specified connection program that seems to be characteristic of central neurons.

Sensory and central neurons differ in other ways. Several years ago, we first showed that crustacean motor axons have a remarkable response to axonotomy. For up to several months following section of the axon, the distal, enucleated fiber will still conduct impulses and release transmitter in normal amounts—even after what should be exhausting tetani containing 100,000 impulses (Hoy, Bittner, and Kennedy, 1967). Observations made in our laboratory, in collaboration with George Bittner, agree with those of Nordlander and Singer (1972) in showing that the distal axons survive but have expanded glial enwrappings.

The mechanisms used by the central stumps of such

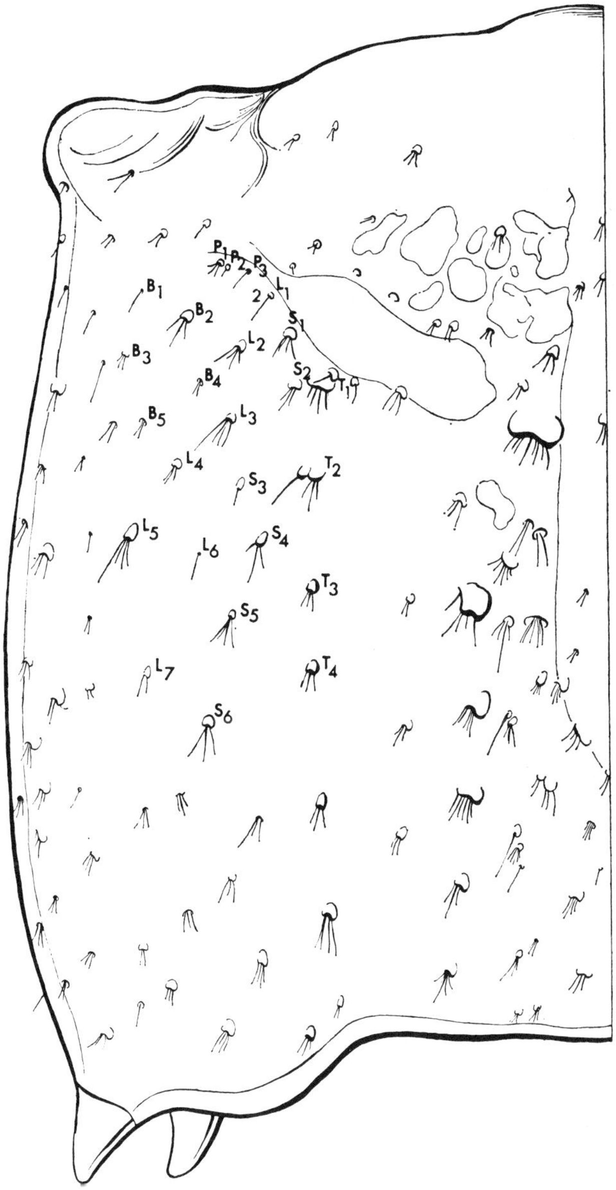

FIGURE 3 Drawing of the exoskeletal hairs in the region of the crayfish telson innervated by root 4 of the sixth ganglion. The hairs make connections with identified interneurons, as analyzed in Figure 4.

axons to reconnect with the muscle are not known. However, our observations, and subsequent ones by Hoy (1969) and by Bittner (unpublished), are consistent with the idea that the outgrowing central axon reconnects with the surviving distal segment. Nordlander and Singer (1972) disagree, primarily on the basis of having seen multiple axonal processes in a region distal to the point at which the cut was made. The matter is not yet resolved; what is clear is that the regeneration is correct, in the sense that outgrowing motor axons reconnect with their own muscles so that adaptive reflex responses are restored.

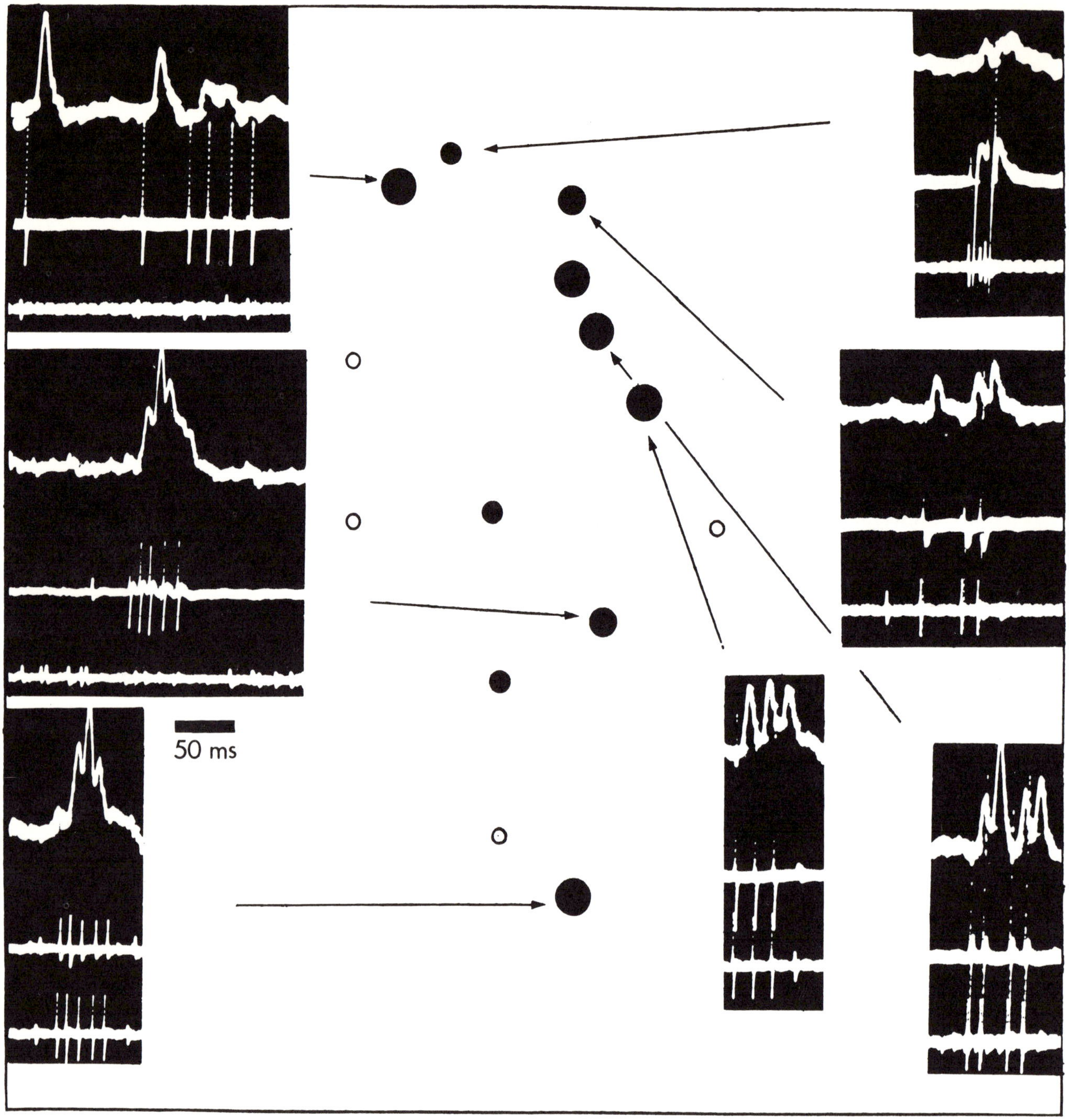

FIGURE 4 Receptive field or "connection" map for sensory hairs in the region shown in Figure 3. *Lower traces:* Proximal and distal *en passant* recordings from the fourth root, sixth ganglion. *Top traces:* Unitary EPSPs recorded from a first-stage interneuron. The size of the spot marking the hair's position reflects the relative amplitude of the first unitary EPSP in a train. For further details see Kennedy (1971).

Central interneurons respond in much the same fashion; they take a very long time to degenerate after sectioning, as has been observed by Wine (1973) for the medial giant axon, and they restore approximately appropriate central connections upon regeneration.

We have now shown, both by electrophysiological tests and by electron microscopy, that sensory neurons behave in an entirely different way. Clear signs of degeneration are apparent in axons separated from their peripherally located cell bodies for two weeks, and after four weeks they are nearly unrecognizable as neurons. Between these times, they lose their capacity to activate other neurons synaptically. Outgrowth of the axons still attached to their perikarya is vigorous, so that limited restoration of function in a crushed root takes place within three weeks.

There is now abundant evidence that these restored connections are appropriate *in a general way*. After severing the sensory nerves to the sixth abdominal ganglion, we find (Kennedy and Wine, work in progress) that tactile afferents make new connections with ascending interneurons even after taking tortuous, ectopic routes into the ganglion. These are roughly correct, in that hairs in the appropriate region of the tail reestablish their normal pattern of contacts upon particular interneurons. Edwards and Sahota (1967) and Edwards and Palka (1971) have shown that regenerating afferents from cricket cerci also reconnect with ascending "giant" interneurons. Here, too, the analysis is relatively coarse: It does not speak to the question of whether particular identified cells reconnect with other specific neurons. Thus we can only conclude that in arthropods the extent of connection specification for sensory fibers relates a peripheral *region* to particular central neurons; as far as we now know, the sensory axons display no more specificity than that during the reconnection process.

In addition to these differences in connection specificity and regeneration patterns, the sensory neurons show another unique feature: They are continually added during life. Crayfish hatch from the egg in nearly the adult form, but with a length of only 5 mm or so. They then undergo a series of molts, at first at intervals of a few days and eventually of weeks or months, that takes them to adult size in one to two years—an increase of about twentyfold in length. As far as we know, the very young animal has a full complement of central and motor neurons—at least all the large and obvious ones can be found. But the periphery is adding new sensory structures all the time: The number of ommatidia in the eye is increasing, more cuticular hairs are being produced, and the number of sensory fibers in peripheral roots is multiplying. Figure 5 gives some values measured on montages prepared from electron micrographs of the fourth root of ganglion 6 (a sensory root) and of the connective between abdominal ganglia 5 and 6. The number of sensory axons increases by nearly tenfold during development.

We now believe that these findings can be applied to the receptive field organization discussed above. Although some addition of new exoskeletal sensory structures takes place between already formed elements, much of it occurs at the lateral and distal margins of the segment. The axons innervating these marginal hairs are small, judging from the amplitudes of their extracellularly recorded impulses.

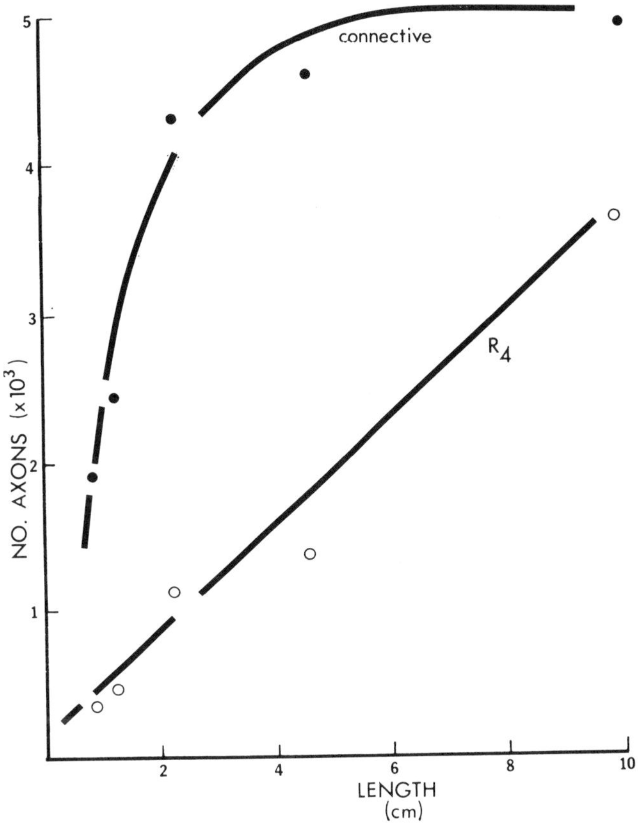

FIGURE 5 Number of axon profiles in the 5–6 connective and the fourth root of the sixth ganglion as a function of size: All points are counts from montages such as that shown in Figure 6.

We suppose that the largest axons belong to the "pioneer" hairs—those that developed earliest. These are also the elements that have the highest probability of connecting with the identified interneurons, though the occasional connections made by axons from the marginal hairs are just as effective as those formed by the larger ones. According to this hypothesis, age both increases cell size (the diameter enlargement is of the order of tenfold for the largest axons) and confers an improved probability that connection will have occurred.

The other curve in Figure 5 makes a separate point that may provide comfort for those of us who believe that arthropod nervous systems hold out some hope for complete circuit analysis. We have all been worried, as Wiersma was in 1952, about the number of fine fibers in the central nervous system. After Cold Spring Harbor, things got worse instead of better: The electron microscope turned up previously uncounted small axons in the central connectives, and the estimates were revised upward (see Figure 6). In young animals, we find that the number of neurons in a 5–6 abdominal connective is only about 1800, as compared with the adult count of 5000. The increase we presume to be due mainly to the addition of sensory axons, and the main difference in the numbers seems to come in several discrete pockets of very small axons (Figures 6 and 7). If these assumptions are correct, we can use the ratios of increase in the sensory roots and in the CNS to estimate the number of sensory axons present in the CNS at hatching. This number turns out to be about 1200 cells, leaving only 600 cells per connective as the complement of "central" neurons.

In several respects, then, the sensory cells have a different biology from the central neurons. The former are epithelial in origin, and thus arise from a continuous source of newly differentiated products. The sensory cells

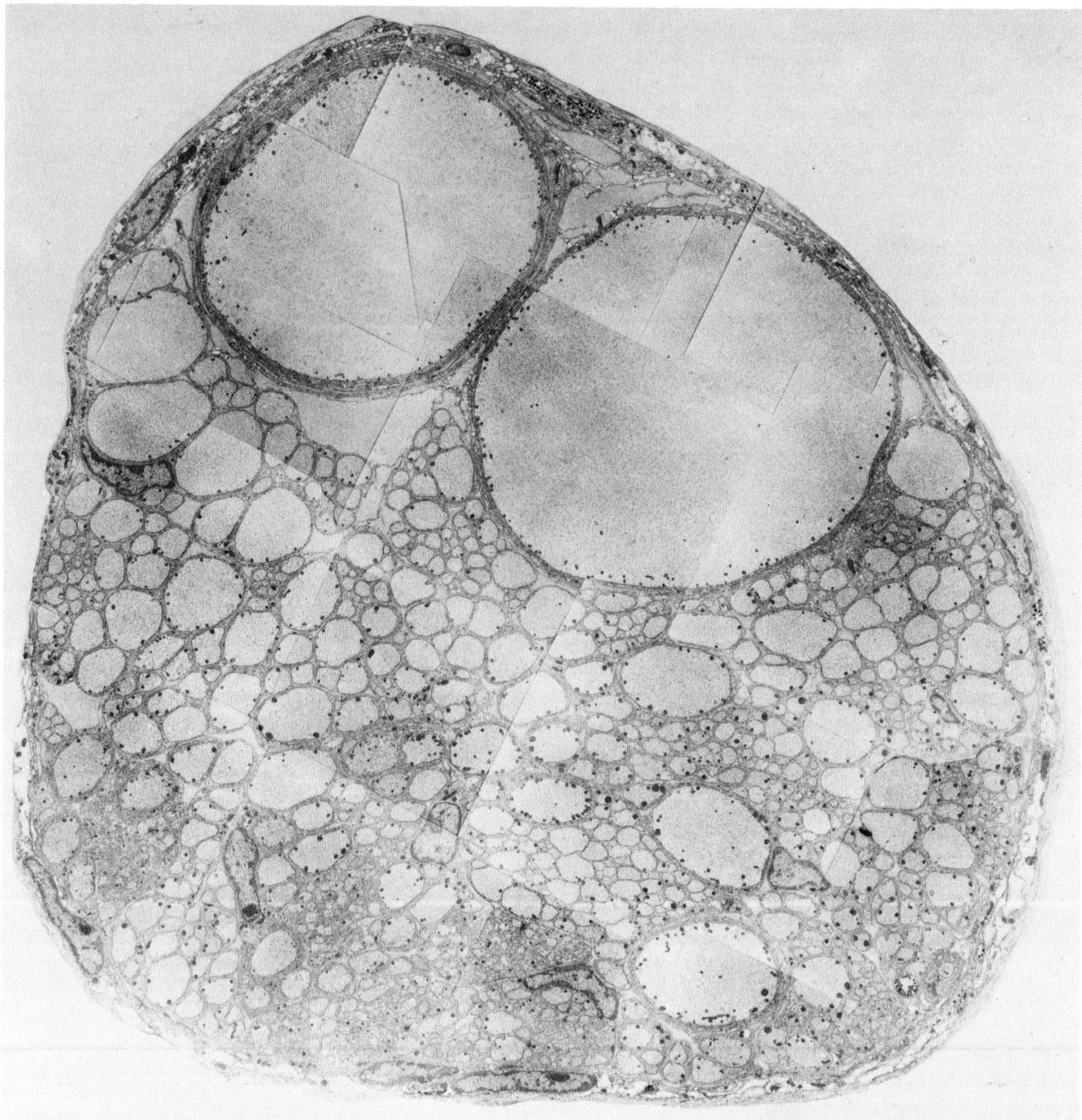

FIGURE 6 Montage of the 5–6 abdominal connective in an approximately fifth-molt animal. The largest axon profile (top right) is the lateral giant; its diameter is approximately 20 μ.

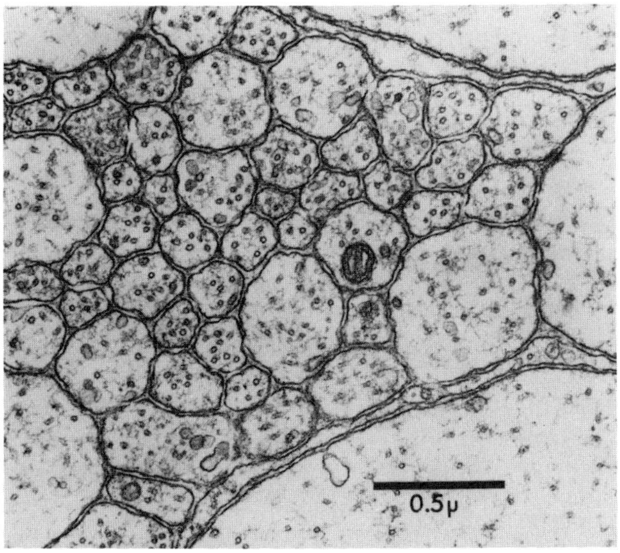

FIGURE 7 Detail of a region of small axons from the 5–6 connective illustrated in Figure 6.

exhibit an "open" developmental history that contrasts with that of the central cells that display fixed number and early specification. Sensory neurons show a much heavier dependence upon the presence of a nucleus and may well regenerate by an entirely different mechanism. Their connections are apparently less individually specified than those of the central elements. (Parenthetically it should be noted that some sensory cells in annelids, molluscs, and certain arthropods have been dealt with as unique, identified cells with individually specified connections. Virtually all of these cases involve neurons having central, rather than peripheral, somata. This important difference suggests that such cells may have originally been central neurons and developed their sensory function secondarily.)

The fixed central elements must adjust continuously to the growth of input provided by the late-developing sensory axons. The duality of the neuronal population raises important questions about the nature of this accommodation. Is late-arriving input concentrated in distal dendritic regions and, hence, less effective? Our experiments to date suggest not. Are the connection probabilities of late-arriving fibers improved by accidental denervation of inputs established earlier? Indeed, are there any alterations in connectivity as a result of derangements in the developmental pattern? We are now taking advantage of the unique identity of the central elements to ask these questions of a second set of nerve cells that, though less unique, may just on that account be more interesting.

ACKNOWLEDGMENT Recent work from the author's laboratory was supported by Grant NB 02944 from the U.S.P.H.S. I acknowledge the help of Joan Misch with the electron microscopy; Joanna Hanawalt provided unflagging technical assistance and criticized this manuscript. I also benefited from helpful discussions with colleagues who deserve mention quite apart from their contributions discussed in the text: Jeffrey Wine, Robert Zucker, Ronald Calabrese, Richard Roth, Jan Letourneau, and Paul Grobstein.

REFERENCES

ASADA, Y., and M. V. L. BENNETT, 1971. Experimental alteration of coupling resistance at an electrotonic synapse. *J. Cell Biol.* 49:159–172.

BARKER, D. L., E. HERBERT, J. G. HILDEBRAND, and E. A. KRAVITZ, 1972. Acetylcholine and lobster sensory neurons. *J. Physiol. (London)*, (in press).

BRUNER, J., and D. KENNEDY, 1970. Habituation: Occurrence at a neuromuscular junction. *Science* 169:92–93.

DAVIS, W. J., and D. KENNEDY, 1972. Command interneurons controlling swimmeret movements in the lobster. I. Types of effects on motoneurons. *J. Neurophysiol.* 35(1):1–12.

EDWARDS, J. S., and J. PALKA, 1971. Neural regeneration: Delayed formation of central contacts in insect sensory cells. *Science* 172:591–594.

EDWARDS, J. S., and T. S. SAHOTA, 1967. Regeneration of a sensory system: The formation of central connections by normal and transplanted cerci of the house cricket *Acheta domesticus*. *J. Exp. Zool.* 166(3):387–396.

EVOY, W. H., and D. KENNEDY, 1967. The central nervous organization underlying control of antagonistic muscles in the crayfish. I. Types of command fibers. *J. Exp. Zool.* 165:223–238.

FIELDS, H. L., 1966. Proprioceptive control of posture in the crayfish abdomen. *J. Exp. Biol.* 44:455–468.

FIELDS, H. L., W. H. EVOY, and D. KENNEDY, 1967. Reflex role played by efferent control of an invertebrate stretch receptor. *J. Neurophysiol.* 30:859–874.

HOY, R. R., 1969. Degeneration and regeneration in abdominal flexor motor neurons in the crayfish. *J. Exp. Zool.* 172(2): 219–232.

HOY, R. R., G. D. BITTNER, and D. KENNEDY, 1967. Regeneration in crustacean motoneurons: Evidence for axonal refusion. *Science* 156:251–252.

KENNEDY, D., 1971. Crayfish interneurons. *The Physiologist* 14: 5 30.

KENNEDY, D., W. H. EVOY, B. DANE, and J. T. HANAWALT, 1967. The central nervous organization underlying control of antagonistic muscles in the crayfish. II. Coding of position by command fibers. *J. Exp. Zool.* 165:239–248.

KENNEDY, D., and J. B. PRESTON, 1960. Complex responses of central neurons in the crayfish to presynaptic and direct stimulation. *Anat. Rec.* 148:360.

KENNEDY, D., A. I. SELVERSTON, and M. P. REMLER, 1969. Analysis of restricted neuronal networks. *Science* 164:1488–1496.

KRASNE, F. B., and CH. A. STIRLING, 1972. Synapses of crayfish abdominal ganglia with special attention to afferent and efferent connections of the lateral giant fibers. *Z. Zellforsch.* 127:526–644.

LARIMER, J. L., A. C. EGGLESTON, L. M. MASUKAWA, and D. KENNEDY, 1971. The different connections and motor outputs of lateral and medial giant fibers in the crayfish. *J. Exp. Biol.* 54:391–402.

LARIMER, J. L., and D. KENNEDY, 1969. The central nervous control of complex movements in the uropods of crayfish. *J. Exp. Biol.* 51:135–150.

NORDLANDER, R. H., and M. SINGER, 1972. Electron microscopy of severed motor fibers in the crayfish. *Z. Zellforsch.* 126: 157–181.

PRESTON, J. B., and D. KENNEDY, 1960. Integrative synaptic mechanisms in the caudal ganglion of the crayfish. *J. Gen. Physiol.* 43:671–681.

REMLER, M. P., A. I. SELVERSTON, and D. KENNEDY, 1968. Lateral giant fibers of crayfish: Location of somata by dye injection. *Science* 162:281–283.

SANDEMAN, D. C., 1969. The site of synaptic activity and impulse initiation in an identified motoneuron in the crab brain. *J. Exp. Biol.* 50:771–784.

SANDEMAN, D. C., and C. M. MENDUM, 1971. The fine structure of the central synaptic contacts on an identified crustacean motoneuron. *Z. Zellforsch.* 119(4):515–525.

SELVERSTON, A. I., and D. KENNEDY, 1969. Structure and function of identified nerve cells in the crayfish. *Endeavour* 27: 105–108.

SELVERSTON, A. I., and M. P. REMLER, 1972. Neural geometry and activation of crayfish fast flexor motorneurons. *J. Neurophysiol.* 35:797–814.

STRETTON, A. O. W., and E. A. KRAVITZ, 1968. Neuronal geometry: Determination with a technique of intracellular dye injection. *Science* 162:132–134.

TAKEDA, K., and D. KENNEDY, 1964. Some potentials and modes of activation of crayfish motoneurons. *J. Cell Comp. Physiol.* 64:165–182.

TAKEDA, K., and D. KENNEDY, 1965. The mechanism of discharge pattern formation in crustacean interneurons. *J. Gen. Physiol.* 48:435–453.

WIERSMA, C. A. G., 1952. Neurons of arthropods. *Cold Spring Harb. Symp. Quant. Biol.* 17:155–163.

WIERSMA, C. A. G., 1958. On the functional connections of single units in the central nervous system of the crayfish, *Procambarus clarkii* (Girard). *J. Comp. Neurol.* 110:421–471.

WIERSMA, C. A. G., and B. M. H. BUSH, 1963. Functional neuronal connections between the thoracic and abdominal cords of the crayfish, *Procambarus clarkii* (Girard). *J. Comp. Neurol.* 121:207–235.

WIERSMA, C. A. G., and G. M. HUGHES, 1961. On the functional anatomy of neuronal units in the abdominal cord of the crayfish, *Procambarus clarkii* (Girard). *J. Comp. Neurol.* 116: 209–228.

WIERSMA, C. A. G., and K. IKEDA, 1964. Interneurons commanding swimmeret movements in the crayfish, *Procambarus clarkii* (Girard). *Comp. Biochem. Physiol.* 12:509–525.

WILSON, D. M., 1970. Neural operations in arthropod ganglia. In *The Neurosciences: Second Study Program*, F. O. Schmitt, ed. New York: Rockefeller University Press, pp. 397–408.

WINE, J., 1973. Invertebrate central neurons: Orthograde degeneration and retrograde changes following axonotomy. *Experimental Neurol.* (in press).

WINE, J., and F. B. KRASNE, 1972. The organization of escape behavior in crayfish. *J. Exp. Biol.* 56:1–18.

ZUCKER, R. S., D. KENNEDY, and A. I. SELVERSTON, 1971. Neuronal circuit mediating escape responses in crayfish. *Science* 173:645–650.

34 Synaptic and Structural Analysis of a Small Neural System

ALLEN I. SELVERSTON and BRIAN MULLONEY

ABSTRACT The functional connectivity patterns in the crayfish fast flexor and the lobster stomatogastric system are constant from animal to animal. Studies utilizing new histological methods indicate that the topology of the individual neurons involved in these motor systems is less consistent. The way in which such anatomical variation can produce functionally equivalent circuits is discussed.

BECAUSE IT HAS been so difficult to determine the detailed circuitry of complex neuronal networks, many neurobiologists have instead sought to analyze their global properties by correlating changes in electrical fields with different behavioral states of the animal. This approach has not been very successful.

If we consider smaller neuronal systems, such as those found in the central nervous systems of some invertebrates, we see that it is neither necessary nor desirable to look for such global properties as EEGs. One can instead describe these systems in terms of the properties of their individual elements and the synaptic relationships between individual elements. Perhaps such a reductionist methodology may never be applicable to the nervous systems of higher animals, because invertebrate nerve cells might somehow differ in their integrative properties. Similarly, a detailed analysis of single invertebrate cells may fail to consider adequately any unique properties of the network as a whole. We take the view that understanding the mechanisms by which small neural networks produce patterned motor output will reveal principles that apply to more complex networks. If all constraints between the nerve cells in a system can be described quantitatively, they can be used effectively to model the system, that is, to describe and predict the output of the whole system. We think that such a component analysis provides an adequate description of the system.

Many nervous systems can generate complex patterns of activity in sets of motor neurons even when isolated completely from all sensory input. Such patterns resemble more or less the patterns associated with particular modes of behavior in the intact animal. We are now close to a description of the mechanisms that generate stereotyped behavior in a few small nervous systems in arthropods, relying heavily on the presence of identifiable neurons.

ALLEN I. SELVERSTON and BRIAN MULLONEY Department of Biology, University of California, San Diego, La Jolla, California

Identifiable neurons

An identifiable neuron is a neuron that can be found in, and that performs the same physiological function in, each individual of a species. Often these neurons exist in bilaterally symmetric pairs, each member being a mirror image of the other with regard to its anatomy. Vertebrate neurons that can be identified as to class—for example, Purkinje cells or motor neurons innervating the extensor digitorum longus—can be reliably assigned as belonging to a particular functional class, but each member cannot reliably be distinguished in different animals. They are not, therefore, identifiable neurons. Identifiable neurons, singly or in combination, permit the experimenter to control experiments properly. Identifiable cells are thus as important to the physiologist as pure chemicals to the molecular biologist.

The stomatogastric ganglion

The stomatogastric ganglion (St G) of the lobster *Panulirus interruptus* generates all the coordinated movements of the animal's stomach. Unlike vertebrates, the stomach of the lobster originates from ectodermal tissue, is lined with chitin, contains no smooth muscle, and has a set of internal teeth that chew food after it enters the stomach. Striated muscles move the stomach, and the motor neurons of the stomatogastric ganglion control their contractions. Early workers (Huxley, 1880; Parker, 1876), in a burst of overenthusiasm for comparative anatomy, gave the various parts of the crustacean stomach names identical to those of the vertebrate stomach; all these homologies are false. Worse, the nervous system that controls the stomachs of Crustacea has been incorrectly homologized with the sympathetic nervous system of vertebrates (e.g., Orlov, 1927). These cumulative errors have produced a nomenclature for the system that obscures reality and misleads the reader but that is firmly established by precedent and has recently been standardized (Maynard and Dando, in preparation).

The St G of *Panulirus* contains about thirty neurons. Twenty-four of these are motor neurons, two are interneurons, and four are of unknown function but have distinctive physiological characteristics. There may also be some sensory neurons (Larimer and Kennedy, 1966); we have not investigated this point. All the neurons are monopolar, and their somata form a cortex around a central neuropil, where all synaptic interactions occur. Unlike many arthropod monopolar neurons, both attenuated spikes and subthreshold synaptic activity can be recorded from their somata. All can be penetrated with microelectrodes under visual control since their somata vary in diameter from about 15 μm to 60 μm.

The isolated St G produces two independent rhythmic motor patterns in discrete sets of motor neurons (Figure 1) (Maynard, 1972). The slower rhythm occurs in motor neurons innervating muscles in the anterior wall of the stomach that move the heavy teeth. These motor neurons form the gastric subsystem of the St G. The faster rhythm occurs in motor neurons that innervate muscles in the posterior pyloric region of the stomach. This region acts as a filter to sort food particles for entry into either the midgut or the hepatopancreas (Yonge, 1924). These neurons form the pyloric subsystem of the St G. The two rhythms can occur simultaneously, or either one can be present in the absence of the other, or both may be absent. The isolated ganglion can change irregularly from one of these operational states to another. In the intact lobster, all four states do occur (Cynthia Mayer, personal communication).

Both rhythms can be modulated by input from the central nervous system. Two unpaired fibers from the supraesophageal ganglion enter the St G via the inferior ventricular nerve and the stomatogastric nerve (SGN). These fibers selectively excite elements of the pyloric subsystem (Dando and Selverston, 1972) and interneuron 1 of the gastric subsystem (Mulloney and Selverston, in preparation). In addition to these two fibers, there are numerous other fibers in the SGN that excite the gastric subsystem (D. K. Hartline, personal communication).

What are the ways by which these motor patterns are generated in the St G? We have recorded the integrative activity of all but one of its cells with intracellular microelectrodes while monitoring extracellularly the activity of all the other neurons. The cells can be positively

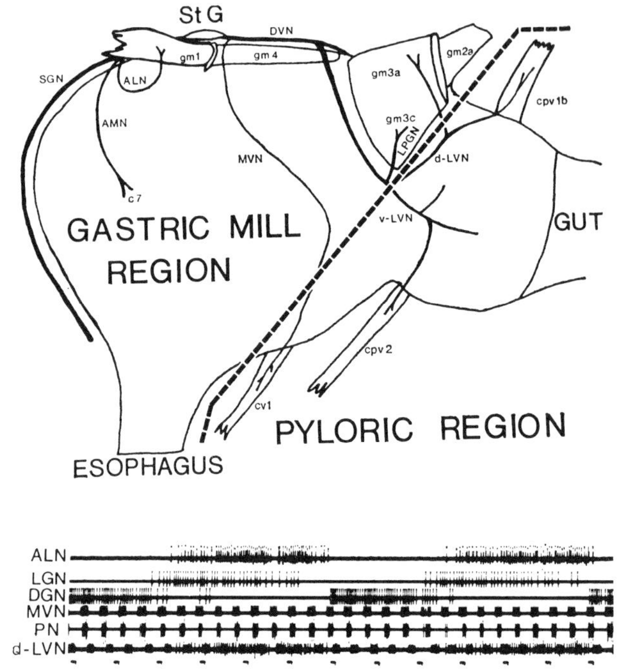

FIGURE 1 *Above:* Side view of lobster stomach. The two principal functional divisions, the gastric mill region and the pyloric region, are separated by a dashed line. Part of the stomatogastric nervous system is shown together with a few of the stomach muscles that they innervate. The stomatogastric ganglion (St G) can be seen on the dorsal surface of the stomach just above gastric mill muscle 1 (gm 1). *Below:* The two basic rhythms produced by the isolated ganglion can be seen in the extracellular recordings from nerves supplying the two different regions of the stomach. The top three nerves (ALN, LGN, DGN), not all shown here, supply muscles that operate the gastric mill. Note that the bursts of activity bear a particular phase relationship with each other and that the duration of each burst lasts several seconds. The three lower traces contain axons of motor neurons (MVN, PN, d-LVN) supplying pyloric muscles. The burst durations are much shorter, and the overall frequency is about seven times as fast as the gastric mill. Note also that the bursts of activity maintain a particular phase relationship. The d-LVN trace contains axons innervating both regions (see above), and the long bursts seen in this trace are from axons to muscle gm 3a. (See Figure 4 for abbreviations.)

identified by antidromic stimulation via the extracellular electrodes and by correlating spikes in the soma with spikes in peripheral nerves. An example of the data obtained is shown in Figures 2 and 3. In these figures the cells are firing spontaneously. When the cells are not firing, synaptic relationships can be ascertained by passing current through one microelectrode while recording simultaneously the intracellular responses of the other cells. The synthesis of such data has produced an almost complete synaptic network diagram for the entire system

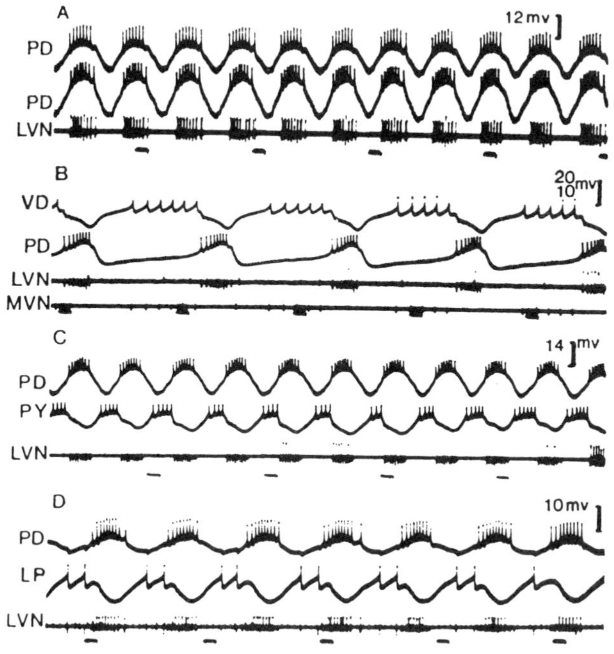

FIGURE 2 Pyloric cycle; intracellular recordings from the somata of pairs of pyloric motor neurons (upper traces) and extracellular recording from the nerves containing the axons (lower traces). (A) Shows the sequential firing of the two PD cells. Note that the spikes occur during the depolarizing phase of the oscillating DC potentials and that the spikes are not locked in 1:1. The occasional large spike in the extracellular trace is from the axon of another motor neuron. (B) Shows the alternation between a PD and a VD cell. (C) Shows alternation between a PD and a PY cell. Only the PD cell is also being recorded extracellularly. (D) Shows the relationship between a PD and a LP cell. Axonal spikes from both units can be seen in the LVN recording. Inhibitory postsynaptic potentials occur in each cell during activity in the other. Time bars are at 1/sec. See text for more details.

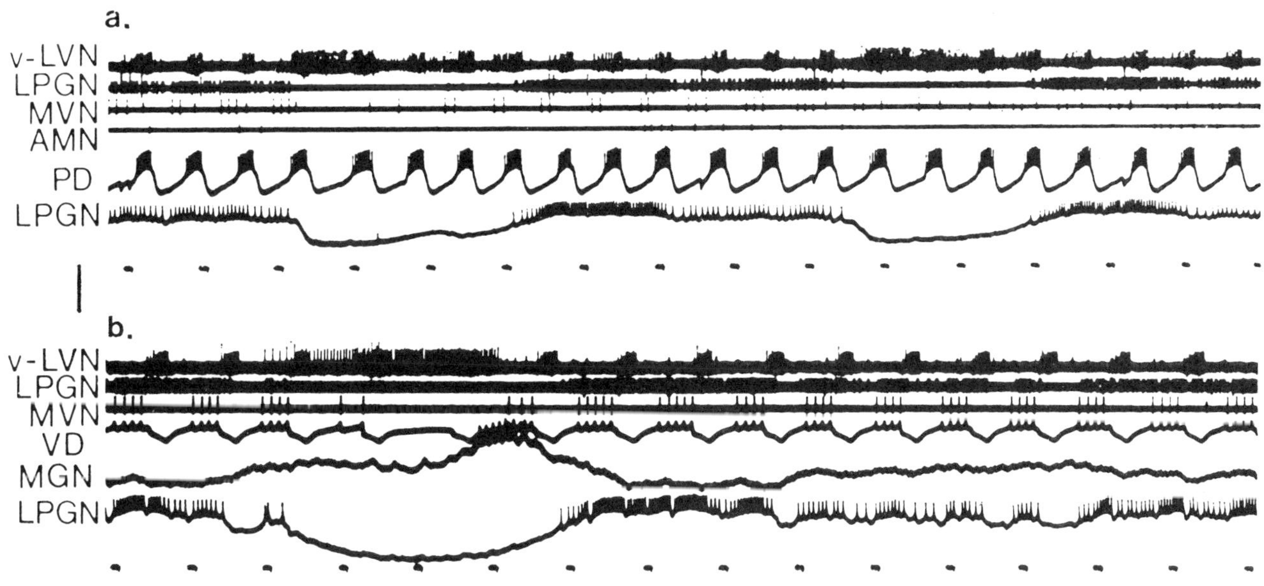

FIGURE 3 Gastric cycle; two examples of recordings from an isolated stomatogastric ganglion, obtained during one experiment. They show alternating bursts between neurons of the gastric system (LPGN, AMN, spikes of LGN, PD, VD, the very large LP spikes on the v-LVN). (a) Shows two intracellular recordings, one from a PD neuron and one from an LPGN. The spikes of each of these neurons were recorded simultaneously on the extracellular traces. The LPGN is alternating with units of the v-LVN trace. The PD is alternating much more frequently with units on the MVN and v-LVN traces. Calibration of intracellular traces: 20 mV. (b) Shows three intracellular traces, one from a VD neuron, whose spikes are also recorded on the MVN trace, one from an MGN, whose spikes are recorded as very small spikes on the v-LVN, and the same LPGN as in (a). During the long burst of spikes on the v-LVN, both the VD and LPGN are inhibited, while the MGN is depolarized and finally fires a short burst. The inhibition of the VD is probably duc to its electrotonic connection with the LPGN. When the LPGN is inhibited, the hyperpolarizing current crosses the electrotonic junction and reduces the firing frequency of the VD. Calibration of intracellular traces: VD, 50 mV; MGN, 10 mV; LPGN, 20 mV. Time marks for both records: 1/sec.

(Figure 4). The network contains 123 inhibitory synapses, 6 chemical excitatory synapses, and 29 electrotonic junctions. The following classes of interactions occur:

1. Unilateral inhibition (DGN and GM)
2. Reciprocal inhibition (MGN and LPGN; VD and IC)
3. Unilateral inhibition with electrotonic coupling (LGN and GM; PD and VD)
4. Reciprocal inhibition with electrotonic coupling (LGN and MGN)
5. Unilateral excitation (Int 2 and Int 1)
6. Electrotonic coupling alone (LPGN and GM)

We have evidence for three additional interactions that we have not yet been able to confirm by simultaneous intracellular recording from the cells involved, and these are not included in Figure 4.

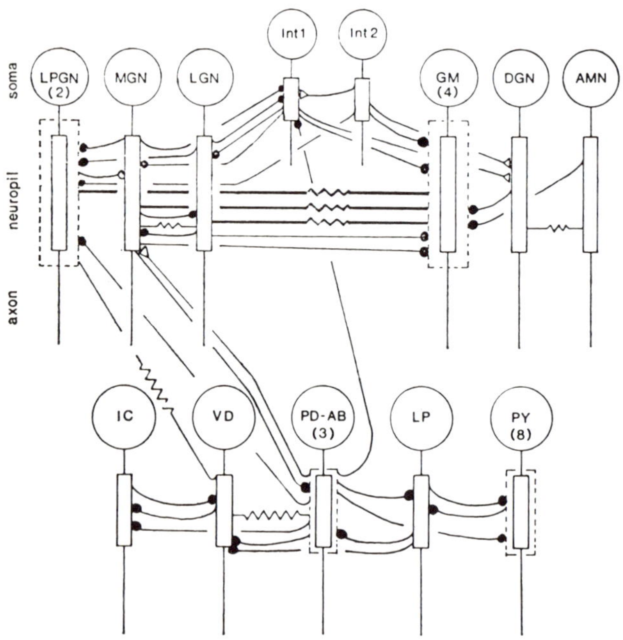

FIGURE 4 Neuronal connectivity diagram for the lobster stomatogastric ganglion. All the cells except Interneurons 1 and 2 are motor neurons. The top ten neurons operate the gastric mill cycle and the bottom fourteen cells operate the pyloric rhythm. The axonal pathways, as well as the muscles innervated by the cells, are known. Soma, neuropile, and axonal parts of the cells are indicated on the left. Dashed lines around some of the neuropile areas indicate that cells of that group are electrotonically connected and can be considered together. Round dots indicate chemical inhibitory synapses; triangles, chemical excitatory synapses; and resistors, electrotonic junctions. Abbreviation of cells indicated in the figure are: LPGN, lateral posterior gastric neuron; MGN, median gastric neuron; LGN, lateral gastric neuron; Int 1 and 2, Interneuron neuron 1 and 2; GM, gastric mill neuron; DGN, dorsal gastric neuron; AMN, anterior median neuron; IC, inferior cardiac; VD, ventricular dilator; PD, pyloric dilator; AB, anterior burster; LP, lateral pyloric; PY, pyloric.

Pyloric rhythm

The network in combination with the properties of the individual neurons explains the observed pattern of motor output in the pyloric subsystem. Like certain neurons in *Aplysia* (Strumwasser, 1965), the PD-AB neurons are endogenous bursters (Maynard, 1972) and determine the periodicity of the pyloric rhythm. The synaptic connections of the neurons in the pyloric subsystem determine the observed pattern. Figure 2 shows examples of intracellular recordings from different cells of the pyloric group.

When the PD-AB group fires, the VD, the LP and the PY cells are all strongly inhibited. After the PD burst the VD and LP cells reach threshold at about the same time even though they are mutually inhibitory. The inhibition from the LP to the PY is stronger, however, so the PY neurons are held below threshold for most of the LP burst, finally firing just before the next PD-AB burst. Each PD-AB burst starts a new cycle.

Gastric rhythm

There is no evidence for the presence of endogenously bursting neurons in this subsystem. The network itself may explain both the periodicity and the pattern of the gastric motor output. The spontaneous output of the ganglion (Figure 3) reflects burst patterns consistent with the synaptic connections.

Preliminary attempts to simulate the gastric network, in collaboration with Donald H. Perkel (Stanford University), show that even without any long time-constant assumptions about the properties of any of the neurons, we are able to get irregular alternating output that resembles remarkably that of the isolated ganglion. The simulated neurons fired regularly, without any bursting, when all synaptic and electrotonic connections were cut. We are now investigating the effects of fatigue and accumulating refractoriness in individual neurons on the stability of the total system.

Pyloric-gastric interactions

At least part of the interactions of the gastric and pyloric rhythms is well explained by the network. When the LGN and MGN fire intense bursts (Figure 3), the VD neuron is strongly inhibited, and the PD-AB neurons are more weakly inhibited. The burst frequency of the PD-AB neurons is decreased temporarily. The electrotonic coupling of the VD and LPGN neurons and the direct inhibition of the MGN onto the PD-ABs explain the results. The LPGNs are strongly inhibited by the LGN and MGN; their somata hyperpolarize some 25 mV when the latter cells fire. This hyperpolarization crosses the electrotonic junction with the VD and inhibits its spontaneous firing. This inhibition can be simulated by passing hyperpolarizing current into the soma of an LPGN; the VD neuron stops firing when the LPGN is hyperpolarized. The PD-ABs are not affected to the same degree by hyperpolarization of the LPGN, but stimulation of the MGN does affect them to an extent comparable to the spontaneous interaction. Discrete synaptic potentials from the MGN are not visible, however, in the PD-AB neurons. The LP neuron is also influenced by the gastric rhythm, but we do not yet know the source of this interaction.

Neuronal structure

The cell bodies in many arthropodan and molluscan ganglia occur in an ordered array. One can often draw a map of the cell bodies and use it to find particular neurons in different animals (Frazier et al., 1967; Otsuka, et al., 1967; Cohen and Jacklet, 1967; Selverston and Remler, 1972). The St G is not organized with this degree of regularity. The soma of a given neuron may be located in any quadrant of the ganglion. We were, therefore, curious to see how much the neuropilar structure of these neurons varied.

Earlier studies of the fast flexor motor neurons in the third abdominal ganglion of *Procambarus clarkii* (Selverston and Remler, 1972), using intracellular recording and injection of Procion dye (Stretton and Kravitz, 1968), showed that both physiological properties and the neuropilar structures of these neurons were very similar in different animals (Figure 5).

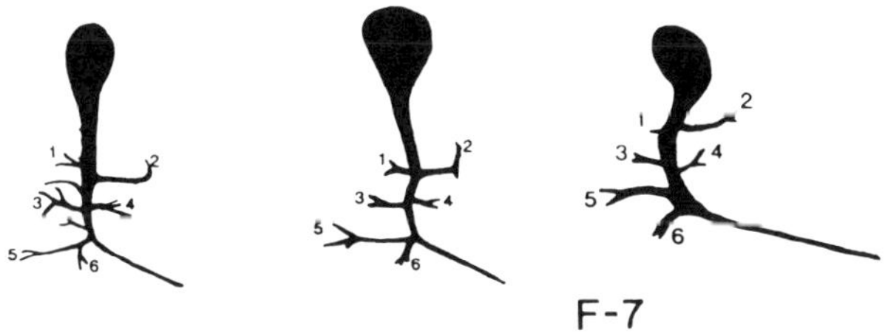

FIGURE 5 Examples of neurons with much more consistent structure can be seen in crayfish abdominal ganglia. Fast-flexor motor neurons have constant cell body locations and similar anatomy. Shown here are tracings from whole mounts of motor neuron F-7 from three different animals. Processes have been numbered and can be compared in each. (For other examples, see Selverston and Remler, 1972.)

The structures of the motor neurons of the St G are much less constant. We have begun to analyze the structural variability of the PD neurons to see if it has physiological significance. The somata of these neurons have no constant location in the ganglion, but their major processes in the neuropil appear similar in each case (Figure 6). The major process leaving the soma bends and descends into the neuropil, bends again and crosses to the other side of the neuropil and finally curves posteriorly and tapers to form the axon. This basic structure is common to all PD neurons (Selverston, 1973). The minor branches of these cells vary both in the point from which they leave the major process and in their orientation in the neuropil. Different PD neurons are not superimposable, even if one compensates for altered orientation of whole mounts. These differences may have no significant effect on the integrative properties of the cells, or some physiological compensation may occur to correct for structural deviation, because the physiological properties of PD neurons are highly consistent in different animals.

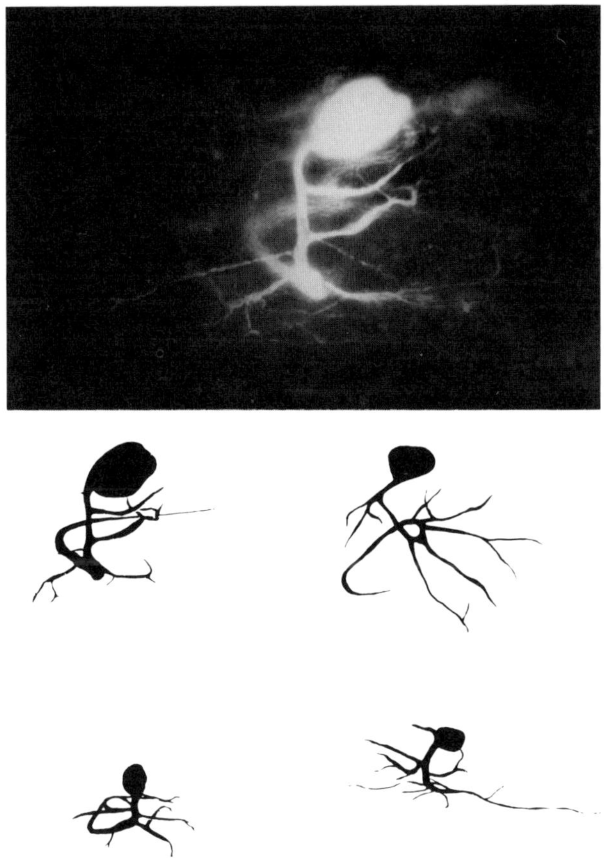

FIGURE 6 A fluorescent whole mount and drawings made from other whole mounts of different PD motoneurons in the stomatogastric ganglion. Although the drawings have been made from different angles of rotation, the basic structure of the cell, as described in the text, is apparent. There is a considerable amount of variation in the smaller processes.

Paired injections

One major test of the network (Figure 4) consisted of injections of Procion dyes into pairs of cells with known physiological interactions. For example, Figure 7a shows

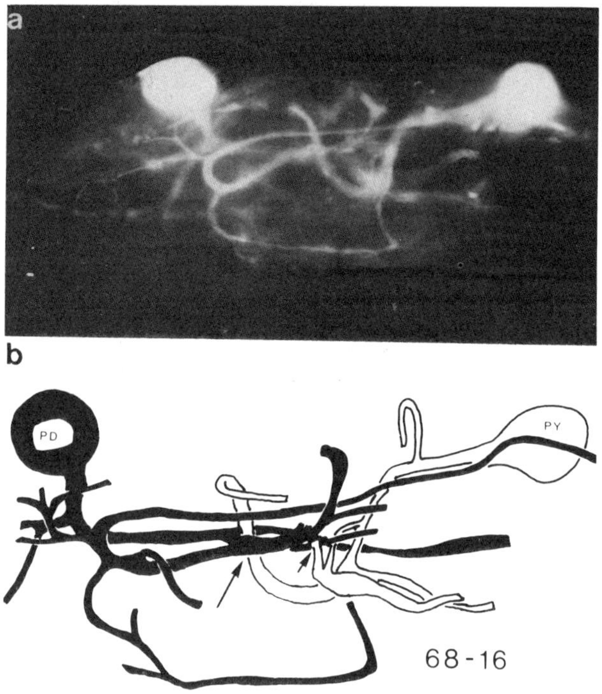

FIGURE 7 The *upper* fluorescent photomicrograph shows a paired Procion yellow injection of two pyloric cycle cells. The PD cell on the left has inhibitory connections to the PY cell on the right. Photographs of paired cells in whole mounts are usually taken from several angles of rotation. The *lower* drawing was made by examining the fluorescent profiles of the sectioned tissue. The arrows indicate points where the processes of the two cells appear to contact one another, and are likely sites of synaptic interaction. (Drawing courtesy of David King.)

a PD and a PY neuron injected with Procion yellow. Figure 7b is a reconstruction of these neurons made by David King (U.C., San Diego) that shows two points of contact between these neurons, as indicated by the arrows. Figure 4 shows only one synaptic interaction between each of the PD and PY neurons. Which of the two points of contact is the synapse whose physiology we know? What is happening at the other point? We do not have enough samples of paired injections of these two cells to answer this question, because it is not possible at the level of light microscopy to identify conclusively the presence and polarity of synapses. New dyes are being developed (see, for example, Pitman, et al., 1972) that will allow us to examine the ultrastructure of such contacts. As we build a library of injected sets of cells, we may be able to assign with certainty the physiological function of an apparent structural contact.

Quantitative analysis of neuronal structure

The traditional methods of reconstructing neurons from serial sections are by the use of stacked sheets of plastic (Selverston and Kennedy, 1969; Mulloney, 1970) and by graphic reconstruction (Pusey, 1939; Iles, 1972). Neither method allows us to measure easily the structural parameters of a cell that are necessary for certain biophysical analyses. Therefore, in collaboration with Sheryl Glasser and N. H. Xuong (U. C., San Diego), we have developed a digital method of reconstructing a neuron from serial sections. The programs permit us to reconstruct and rotate a neuron in three dimensions and to measure accurately cell volume, surface area, the power relations and numbers of branch points, lengths of processes, and other parameters of this sort. This information combined with physiological data from the same cell may allow us to model and understand the integrative processes of these neurons with considerable accuracy.

Summary

We have described virtually the entire network of synaptic connections in the stomatogastric ganglion of *Panulirus interruptus*. This network explains in part the patterned firing of the motor neurons in the ganglion.

Structural evidence obtained with intracellular dyes corroborates the physiological results.

ACKNOWLEDGMENTS The authors' research is supported by grants number NS-09322 and NS-10629 from N.I.H. and by the Alfred P. Sloan Foundation. Brian Mulloney is a post-doctoral fellow of NINDS-NIH.

REFERENCES

COHEN, M. J., and J. W. JACKLET, 1967. The functional organization of motor neurons in an insect ganglion. *Phil. Trans. Roy. Soc. (London)* 252(B):501–527.

DANDO, M. R., and A. I. SELVERSTON, 1972. Command fibers from the supraoesophageal ganglion to the stomatogastric ganglion in *Panulirus argus*. *J. Comp. Physiol.* 78:138–175.

FRAZIER, W. T., E. R. KANDEL, I. KUPFERMANN, R. WAZIRI, and R. E. COGGESHALL, 1967. Morphological and functional properties of identified neurons in the abdominal ganglion of *Aplysia californica*. *J. Neurophysiol.* 30:1288–1351.

HUXLEY, T. H., 1880. *The Crayfish: An Introduction to the Study of Zoology*. London: Kegan Paul and Co.

ILES, J. F., 1972. Structure and synaptic activation of the fast coxal depressor motor neuron of the cockroach *Periplaneta americana*. *J. Exp. Biol.* 56:647–656.

LARIMER, J. L., and D. KENNEDY, 1966. Visceral afferent signals in the crayfish stomatogastric ganglion. *J. Exp. Biol.* 44:345–354.

MAYNARD, D. M., 1972. Simpler networks. *Ann. N.Y. Acad. Sci.* 193:59–72.

MULLONEY, B., 1970. The structure of the giant fibers of earthworms. *Science* 168:994–996.

ORLOV, J., 1927. Das Magenganglion des Fluszkrebses. *Z. Mikr. Anat. Forsch.* 8:73–96.

OTSUKA, M., E. A. KRAVITZ, and D. D. POTTER, 1967. Physiological and chemical architecture of a lobster ganglion with particular reference to GABA and glutamate. *J. Neurophysiol.* 30:725–752.

PARKER, T. J., 1876. On the stomach of the freshwater crayfish. *J. Anat. Physiol.* (quoted in Huxley, T. H., 1880).

PITMAN, R. M., C. D. TWEEDLE, and M. J. COHEN, 1972. Branching of central neurons: Intracellular cobalt injection for light and electron microscopy. *Science* 176:412–414.

PUSEY, H. K., 1939. Methods of reconstruction from microscope sections. *J. Roy. Microsc. Soc.* 59:232–244.

SELVERSTON, A. I., 1973. The use of intracellular dye injections in the study of small neural networks. In *Intracellular Staining Techniques in Neurobiology*, S. Kater, and C. Nicholson, eds. New York: Springer-Verlag (in press).

SELVERSTON, A. I., and D. KENNEDY, 1969. Structure and function of identified nerve cells in the crayfish. *Endeavour* 38: 107–114.

SELVERSTON, A. I., and M. P. REMLER, 1972. Neural geometry and activation of crayfish fast flexor motorneurons. *J. Neurophysiol.* (in press).

STRETTON, A. O. W., and E. A. KRAVITZ, 1968. Neuronal geometry: Determination with a technique of intracellular dye injection. *Science* 162:132–135.

STRUMWASSER, F., 1965. The demonstration and manipulation of a circadian rhythm in a single neuron. In *Circadian Clocks*, J. Aschoff, ed. Amsterdam: North Holland, pp. 442–462.

YONGE, C. M., 1924. Studies on the comparative physiology of digestion. 2. The mechanism of feeding, digestion, and assimilation in *Nephrops norvegicus*. *J. Exp. Biol.* 1:343–389.

35 Neural Machinery Underlying Behavior in Insects

GRAHAM HOYLE

ABSTRACT Neuron somata of large insects, especially locusts, are being impaled with microelectrodes in preparations that permit movements of limbs. Motor neurons are identified and mapped after physiological testing and Procion dye injection. They are anatomically prescribed and can be relocated by reference to maps. Larger interneurons are also being studied, and by combining recordings from pairs of neuron somata with peripheral recording, the neural bases of integration and of control of locomotion are being examined. An identified tonic motor neuron is being entrained by computer to fire at significantly higher or lower rates than its normal average and the possible physiological basis of the change tested.

THE MAJOR AIM OF this chapter will be to try to show that after a late start insects are about to come into their own as major targets for neuroethological research. Only after the introduction of the fruit fly as a research subject and the concentration of effort on it by a large number of investigators was genetics revolutionized and put on a firm scientific foundation. It is all too obvious that a comparable target for attention is needed in neurobiology. Although the crayfish has been suggested as the standard (Wiersma, 1959), I feel that the subject eventually chosen will be an insect, for some of the same reasons that *Drosophila* is so useful in genetics. A major reason for the delay in using insects in research was the lack of success encountered in many early attempts to record intracellularly from insect ganglia. Within the last three years, however, several investigators have been able to break this barrier and, while it is regrettable that the nervous system of *Drosophila* itself is too small, electrophysiological analysis at levels down to, and including, individual neurons is now possible in larger insects. The great promise offered by insects is because of the likelihood that their behavior, both instinctive and learned, may be amenable to ultimate analysis in terms of underlying neuronal events.

This analysis requires a synthesis starting with ethology for accurate description of an act of behavior and breaking that behavior down into components that are ultimately sequences of muscular contractions and relaxations. Next there should be physiology, if such a distinction needs to be made in view of Wigglesworth's (1939) perceptive, though little known, dictum that "behavior is physiology." Closely correlated with the physiology should be anatomy —the elucidation of the neural circuitry, with attendant synaptology, and its development, especially those experimental approaches aimed at understanding neuronal specificity. Then there should be genetic analysis, to be closely coupled with the foregoing; finally there should be an evolutionary synthesis, relating behaviors in allied species and considering how they may have evolved and be evolving. The available methods will first be considered briefly and then the progress being made in each major category presented.

GRAHAM HOYLE Department of Biology, University of Oregon, Eugene, Oregon

Methods for insect neuroethology

ELECTROMYOGRAMS Insect muscles are operated by a system completely different from that occurring in higher vertebrates, and while this may be a disadvantage from the point of view of transferring knowledge from one area to the other, the simplicity of the insect system offers a great experimental advantage (Figure 1). Many of their muscles are operated by a single motor neuron that innervates each muscle fiber at many points (multiterminal innervation). Tension is varied by altering the frequency of firing. Only a few muscles comprise more than one motor unit. When a second excitatory neuron sharing innervation of the same muscle fibers is present, it gives larger twitch contractions and is used only to boost the peak tension for extra-fast movements (Figure 1B; Hoyle, 1964; Pearson, 1972). The result is that the electromyogram is a digital sequence that is easily recorded and that can be studied quantitatively and from which the resulting movements, though not recorded, can be inferred (Hoyle, 1957). The situation is complicated, for some muscles, by an additional axon or axons of inhibitor type that cause peripheral polarization, but the functional role of these axons is obscure at the present time. They produce only very small, if any, myograms.

The myograms are obtained simply by attaching very

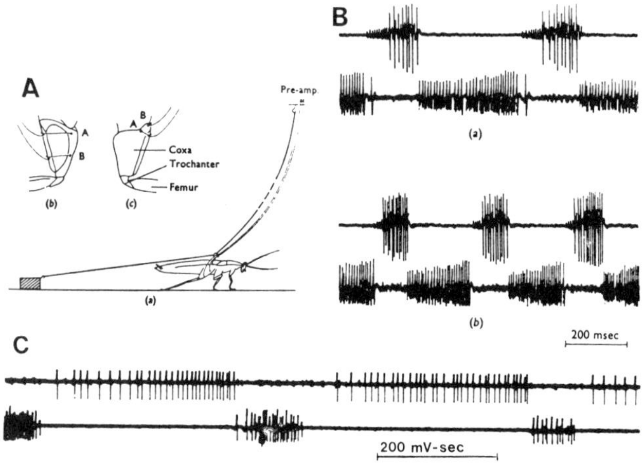

FIGURE 1 (A) Electromyographic method illustrated. (a) Experimental arrangement for recording activity in coxal levator and depressor muscles of a cockroach during walking. The insect's movements were restricted by a fine thread attached to a ring inserted through the dorsal cuticle and to an elevated support in the center of the area. Retraction of the hind legs was resisted by a sliding weight attached to the back. (b) Ventral view of the coxa showing the arrangement of electrodes for recording the depressor activity. (c) Dorsal view of the coxa showing positions for recording the levator activity. (B) Typical electromyograms from antagonists during walking at two different speeds; (a) slow, (b) fast. *Upper traces*: levator (182C) and *bottom traces*: depressor (177D). Discharge in depressor is due to single slow axon giving train of facilitating spikes. Electrical activity in levator includes single slow axon (small, facilitating responses) and single fast axon (large spikes). (C) Recording of spontaneously generated motor nerve spikes going to antagonistic muscles after total removal of leg receptors. Reciprocal output patterns are still present, although at rather low rates. *Upper trace*: levator; *lower trace*: depressor. From Pearson (1972).

fine insulated wires to the insect, with cut ends inserted through the cuticle into the relevant muscles. Larger insects can behave normally while trailing many such leads. The present maximum obtained by Elsner (1968) on a small grasshopper, is 15 pairs of wires. All neurobehavioral studies have used this method, specifically to examine insect flight (reviewed by Wilson, 1968), cricket singing (reviewed by Huber, 1971), grasshopper courtship (reviewed by Elsner, 1973), and cricket and locust walking (Bentley, 1969a; Hoyle, 1964). Wires can also be used to record nerve impulse activity. By correlating nerve and muscle activity in a freely walking locust, Runion and Usherwood (1966) were able to identify inhibitor nerve discharges. They made a check on the efficacy of timing of inhibitor impulses in causing increased relaxation rate by using tape-recorded discharges of the neurons obtained from free-walking preparations in order to excite the axons in slave preparations from which the tension was recorded (Usherwood and Runion, 1970).

MICROELECTRODE RECORDINGS In 1956 two papers reporting extremely promising results for insect neurophysiology were published. Hagiwara and Watanabe (1956) obtained 60 mV resting potentials with glass capillary electrodes placed in the motorneurons of the sound-evoking tymbal muscle of a cicada. Furthermore, as a response to a single afferent volley evoked in the auditory nerve, they could make the neurons fire bursts closely resembling the natural output causing sounds. Spikes were larger than 70 mV, overshooting, and preceded by excitatory postsynaptic potentials (EPSPs) that were sometimes below threshold in size. Maynard (1956), also using a capillary electrode and going straight to the highest place, a cockroach brain, obtained a sharp spike of 30 mV amplitude from the calyx of the corpora pendunculata following electrical stimulation of the antennal nerve. In spite of the size of the response, Maynard stated it was recorded not intracellularly but extracellularly. Several investigators had already tried microelectrodes in insect ganglia and obtained only resting potentials, with no synaptic or spike activity apparent. Stimulated by the above publications, they tried again but with indifferent results. Hagiwara and Watanabe were not sure from which part of the motorneurons they had recorded, nor were they able to extend their work to interneurons. No further progress was reported until 1960 when Rowe (1960) announced briefly that he had recorded inhibitory postsynaptic potentials (IPSPs) as well as EPSPs from a cockroach third thoracic ganglion. Later, after the kind of delay that has beset the subject, Rowe (1969) published pictures of spikes as well as synaptic activity; but since he did not attempt to identify those neurons, his results did not greatly promote the subject. In the preceding year Kerkut, Pitman, and Walker (1968) obtained EPSPs, IPSPs, and overshooting spikes from what was undoubtedly a cell body of the cockroach sixth abdominal ganglion. They used the preparation (Kerkut et al., 1969) to show that the neuron is excited by 1.3×10^{-13} mole acetylcholine and hyperpolarized by 1.05×10^{-13} mole gamma-aminobutyric acid.

Extensive explorations with intracellular electrodes in the mesothoracic ganglion of the cricket (*Gryllus campestris*) were made by Bentley (1969a) who obtained synaptic and spike activity of enormous variety. Some of this was evoked by stimulation of an evasion response; other activity was associated with ventilation and flight. But while showing that insect nervous systems could yield their secrets, the recordings were still not from identified neurons and therefore not sufficient to provide a firm foundation for detailed analysis of any of these activities. Bentley made remarkably fine use of a single preparation of a male cricket that, after localized brain lesions, sang continually for 12 hours. By combined intracellular recording from the ganglion, from unknown, chance sites, and nerve trunks, he obtained recordings of interesting, large prepotentials leading to motor output to specific wing muscles. Many of these were probably from motorneuron somata. He also obtained the first direct evidence of electrical coupling between wing motorneurons.

Meanwhile, the systematic study of both the anatomical and physiological characteristics of the same neuron was made possible by the introduction of the first useful intracellularly injectable dye, Procion Yellow (Stretton and Kravitz, 1968). Hoyle and Burrows (1970; 1973a, b; Burrows and Hoyle, 1973) worked on the motorneurons of the locust third thoracic ganglion (Figure 2) and Bentley (1970) on the flight motorneurons of the locust second thoracic ganglion. Some large neurons on the dorsal surface of the locust and cockroach third thoracic ganglia were added to the list (Crossman et al., 1971) but were not functionally identified, and a few possible premotor interneurons of locusts were located and given preliminary identification by Hoyle and Burrows (1973a, b). Of these the smallest is just less than 20 μm in diameter. The ability to work with neurons of this diameter brings

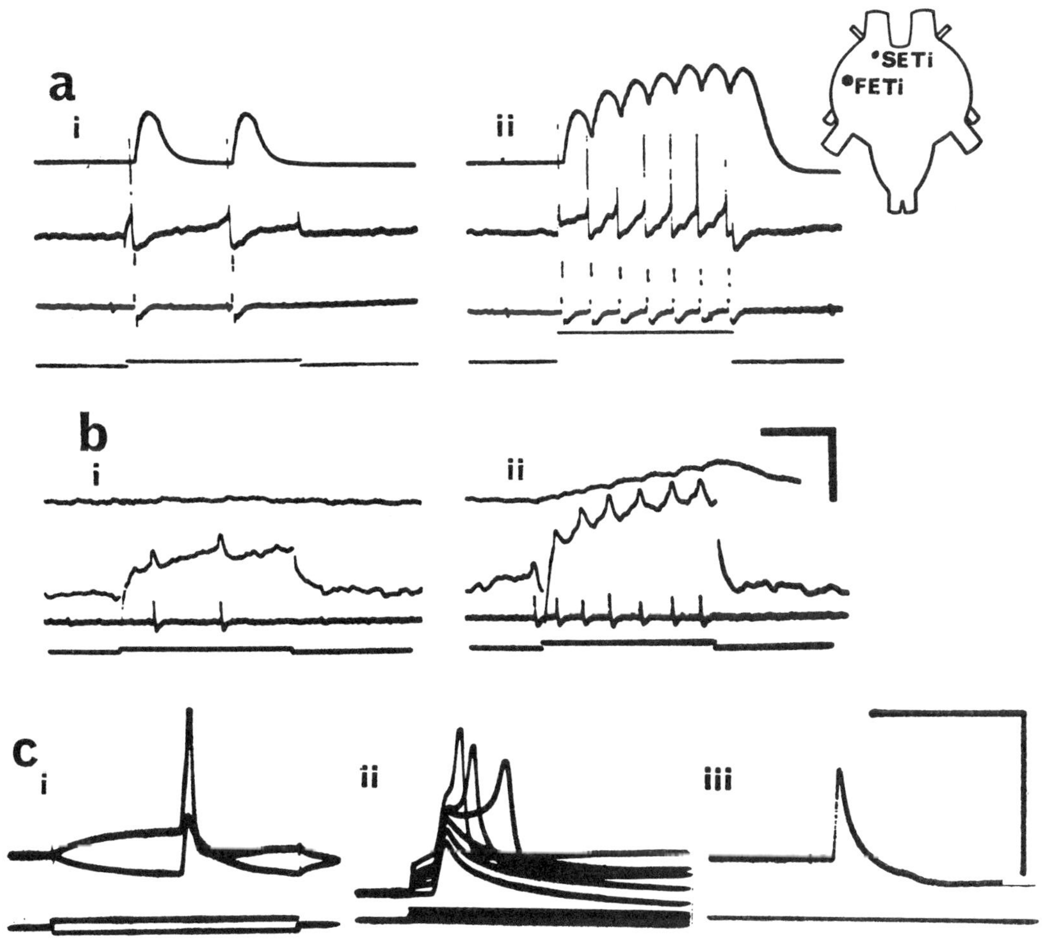

FIGURE 2 Identification of motorneurons and analysis of responses. An intracellular electrode is placed in a suspected motorneuron soma and a depolarizing current pulse passed across it through the microelectrode using a bridge circuit (current monitored on lowest traces) until the cell fires (second traces). Extracellular recordings are made from muscles until the correct one is found (third traces). Confirmation is made by attaching the muscle to a tension recorder (top traces). Locations of motorneurons indicated in insert. (a) i and ii: fast extensor tibiae at two current strengths. (b) i and ii: slow extensor tibiae at two current strengths. Calibration (a) and (b): vertical 10 mV, horizontal 20 msec. (c) Analysis of excitability and response of fast neuron soma. Responses obtained by antidromic excitation. (i) and (ii) With slight hyperpolarization the response is slightly depressed but with slight depolarization it is enhanced. The enhancement is clearly due to the initiation of a graded electrogenic response, probably in the soma membrane. The initial antidromic response is purely electrotonic invasion from the principal neurite. (iii) Antidromic response at normal membrane potential. There is no, or very little, depolarizing electrogenesis, but a large undershoot indicates that strong repolarizing electrogenesis has been initiated. Calibration: 20 mV; (i) and (ii): 40 mse·· (iii) 20 msec. From Hoyle and Burrows (1973a).

within range of experimental manipulation probably all of the motorneurons and about 25% of the interneurons of the locust. Preparations studied range from isolated ganglia, as used by Crossman et al. (1971), to nearly intact preparations. Hoyle and Burrows (1973a, b) used a preparation with the insect on its back, which permitted free movements of the legs but from an unnatural posture. In a preparation recently developed by Dagan and Hoyle, the ganglia are approached from the dorsal surface and the insect is able to assume a normal posture and to walk on a light turntable.

Each experiment is performed with a dye-filled electrode so that an anatomical study can be subsequently made. After fixation, ganglia are photographed before serial sections are made. Projections of these sections are made onto acetate sheets, that on stacking with appropriate spacing, make the reconstructed neuron, with its neurites and dendrites, visible in three dimensions. The fine branches of a neuron are much more clearly seen in whole mounts when filled with cobalt sulfide rather than Procion Yellow. But for three-dimensional reconstruction, the fluorescent dye is easier to use. However, the very finest branches of nerves are not visible. Each specific neuron occupies about the same site in different ganglia and has a similar dendritic topography. It has thus become possible to draw neuron soma location and neurite pathway maps (Figure 3) that are directly useful in further work. For instance, after preparing the map locations, simultaneous recordings from selected pairs of neurons became possible (Hoyle and Burrows, 1973b).

To provide preliminary classification of neuron types located, I shall refer to neurons within the ganglia as either motorneurons, peripheral inhibitor neurons, premotor neurons, sensory integrating interneurons, and all others as other interneurons. Only motorneurons causing excitatory junctional potentials in muscle fibers were thereby easy to define unequivocally. A neuron that makes direct synaptic contact with a motorneuron but has no axonal branch leaving the ganglion will be termed a premotor interneuron. All neurons that receive synaptic input directly from a sense organ and that are not motorneurons or peripheral inhibitors will be termed sensory integrating interneurons. Interneurons that receive input only from these interneurons, or ones of a still higher order that are not also premotor, will be simply termed interneurons.

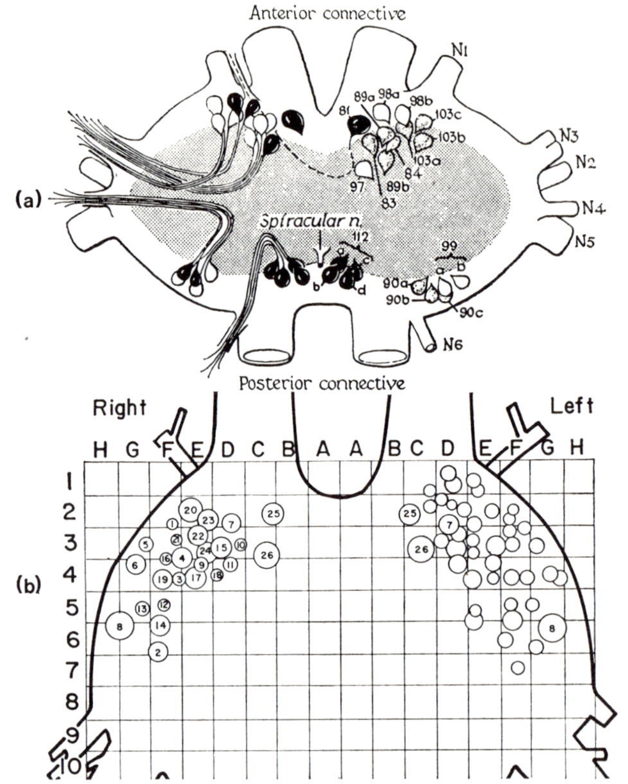

FIGURE 3 Locations of identified neurons of locust (*Schistocerca gregaria*) ganglia. *Upper:* Mesothoracic ganglion indicating flight motorneurons. Numbers refer to muscles innervated. From Bentley (1970). *Lower:* Metathoracic ganglion indicating leg motorneurons with diameters drawn to correct relative scale. Identifications as given on accompanying Table I. Identifications by Burrows and Hoyle (Burrows and Hoyle, 1973; Hoyle and Burrows, 1973a, b; unpublished).

Electrophysiology of insect neurons

The only insect nerve fibers that have been examined in detail electrophysiologically are the "giant" axons of the ventral nerve cord of the cockroach. These axons taper gradually from 30–60 μ to 20–30 μ as they pass from their origin in the last abdominal ganglion, and they also have an abrupt "waist" within each ganglion they pass through (Spira et al., 1969). They have conventional squid-axon type sodium-potassium overshooting spikes that are blocked by tetrodotoxin (Narahashi, 1965); this is probably true of insect axons in general.

The somata, by contrast, are not only unconventional electrically, they have been found to have a wide variety of responses. Even allowing for the possibility of damage during dissection, sheath removal (where involved), loss of tracheal supply, less than optimal bathing solutions, etc., some of the response types observed must be valid ones, because these same factors are common to the same neurons in all experiments. The membranes of neuron somata of insects range, within a single ganglion, from completely electrically inexcitable through weakly to strongly graded electrogenesis to all-or-none spike responsiveness. The latter groups will be dealt with separately.

TABLE I

Identified motorneurons of the metathoracic ganglion of Schistocerca gregaria. *Numbers of muscles are from Albrecht (1953) adapted from Snodgrass*

Muscle	Number	Type	Maximum Soma Diameter Microns (μm)	Identification No.	Grid Reference (all on right side of animal)
Retractor unguis	139a	slow	35	1	F2
		fast	65	2	F7
Levator tarsus	137	slow	40	3	F4
		fast	60	4	E3
Depressor tarsus	138	slow	45	5	G3
		fast	55	6	G4
Extensor tibiae	135	slow	55	7	D2
		fast	90	8	G6
Flexor tibiae	136	Anterior Group			
		slow	40	9	E4
		intermediate	35	10	D3
		fast	45	11	D4
		Posterior Group			
		slow	35	12	F5
		intermediate	45	13	G5
		fast	65	14	F6
Depressor trochanteris	133	fast	65	15	D3
Abductor coxa	125	slow	35	16	F4
		fast	55	17	E4
Adductor coxa	130	slow	35	18	D4
Anterior rotator coxa	121	slow	55	19	F4
		fast	75	20	E2
Posterior rotator coxa	122	slow	30	21	F3
		fast	55	22	E3
Tergosternal	113	fast	70	23	E2
Promotor tergum	118	fast	65	24	E3
Promotor extensor of hind wing (basalar)	128	fast	70	25	C2
Depressor extensor of hind wing (subalar)	29	fast	80	26	C3

ALL-OR-NONE SPIKES In the cockroach sixth abdominal ganglion (Kerkut et al., 1969), all-or-none spikes were recorded in unidentified somata, which may be sensory integrating interneurons of the phallic region. All-or-none spikes were also found in a group of seven or eight unpaired neurons located in the midline on the dorsal surface of locust and cockroach metathoracic ganglia (Crossman et al., 1971). These neurons branch equally to left and right sides and have axons that leave the ganglion in nerve 5, but again their function is unknown. Dagan and Hoyle (in preparation) determined in the locust that they are efferent neurons, although they do not innervate any leg muscles. They are either neurosecretory or innervate a peripheral sensory structure such as a chordotonal organ. Resting potentials in Hoyle's (1953) saline are 50 to 60 mV, overshoots are up to 20 mV, and undershooting after-potentials as much as 25 mV (Figure 4Ai). The height of the total excursion, from peak overshoot to peak undershoot, is constant and about 85 mV when the neuron fires after a rest, but the height wanes rapidly upon repetition, and after a few seconds of firing at a high rate the spike ceases. Both the progressive decay in response and

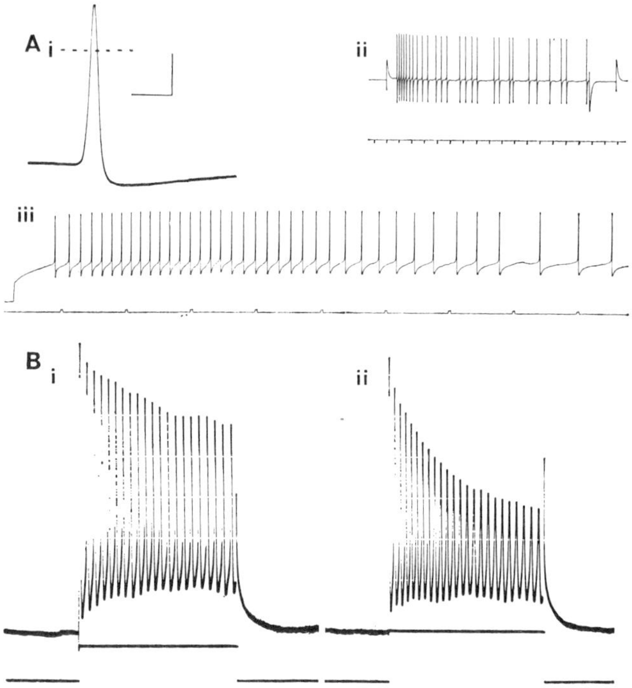

FIGURE 4 Examples of neurons giving overshooting spikes as recorded in the somas. (A) A large, dorsal, unpaired neuron of locust metathoracic ganglion. (i) Single impulse, 90 mV peak to trough, with a 25 mV overshoot from approximate 55 mV resting potential. Spike duration about 8 msec. Calibration: vertical, 20 mV; horizontal, 10 msec. (ii) Slow train from (i) with decreasing frequency initiated by directly applied depolarizing current through overbalanced bridge circuit. Time in seconds. (iii) Fastest train obtainable from (i), in response to break from large hyperpolarizing current pulse. Maximum firing rate 6 Hz. Time in seconds. (B) i and ii: Discharge trains in sensory integrating neuron of locust (auditory) to depolarizing pulses of different strengths for comparison with Figure 4A. Spike duration about 2 msec. Maximum firing rate 300 Hz. Figure 4A from Dagan and Hoyle (in preparation); Figure 4B from Hoyle and Burrows (unpublished).

the early block could be accounted for if these neurons have a tight sheath across which only limited ionic exchange is possible, but there is no evidence for this. The interneuronal space is very slight, with no more than a few millimicrons between axons, which should lead to a rapid local accumulation of potassium. A neuron excited by direct depolarization or by break from hyperpolarization of its soma still fires impulses, but these invade the soma only electrotonically. By additional depolarization soma spikes can still be elicited, but it is a property of these neurons that the electrically excitable response fatigues very rapidly. Nothing is yet known about the ionic permeability mechanisms underlying the spikes. Preliminary studies by Hoyle and Burrows (unpublished) indicate that sensory integrating interneurons, by contrast, fire all-or-none spikes at high rates, with little accommodation (Figure 4B).

GRADED RESPONSES In some large motorneurons of the locust, a spike of up to 30 mV magnitude appears in the soma after an impulse has occurred in the axon following either orthodromic or antidromic excitation. The response is probably antidromically initiated in both cases, because the threshold for firing an action potential in the impulse initiation zone, situated in neuropil some distance from the soma, is very low compared with that of the soma membrane. The response magnitude is fairly constant although it is of graded type, i.e., proportional to the stimulus strength. Its constancy reflects only the all-or-none aspect of the spike that initiates it by electrotonic invasion. If the latter fails to excite depolarizing electrogenesis because it is too weak, it nevertheless usually initiates some repolarizing electrogenesis, causing the electrotonic potential to undershoot. A small depolarizing pulse applied to the soma at the time of invasion leads to activation of such depolarizing electrogenesis (Figure 2c).

Developmental biology of insect nervous systems

In order to understand the nature of neural circuitry in general, it may be essential to follow its development. The use of degeneration and regeneration techniques will also continue to be of great importance as they have in mammals for over a hundred years. In those regards insects are more amenable to experiment than other forms. A wealth of information already exists on the developmental anatomy of insect nervous systems (Edwards, 1969). Now, as it becomes possible to work out the definitive circuitry in parts of adult insect nervous systems, it will be extremely fruitful to correlate developmental and adult regeneration studies with cellular studies.

Two pioneering studies deserve special mention, both on crickets. Edwards and Sahota (1967) found that the sensory nerve fibers of abdominal cerci regenerating after ablation establish normal functional connections with the giant fiber system in the terminal ganglion. This provides a superb model system for testing Sperry's (1943) hypothesis of neuronal specificity. In ganglia deprived of cercal afferents by ablation (Edwards and Palka, 1971), the functional connections are remade, and both the physiological and the behavioral responses can be studied directly. Both were identical to normal, even when the cricket had been deprived of the cercal input from both cerci throughout development.

These results seem to indicate an independent genetic control of the sensory system and the interneuron system (also, see chapter by Kennedy earlier in this part for similar indications in Crustacea), and Edwards pointed out that they appear to contrast strongly with the implications of the well-known findings of Wiesel and Hubel (1963, 1965) on kittens deprived of visual input that the development of the nervous system is dependent upon normal sensory inflow, especially in early stages. But it is compatible with the even more famous optic nerve regeneration experiments of Weiss (review, 1950) and Sperry (1943) on amphibia. There is one major difference technically in that in the Wiesel/Hubel experiments the nerves were not cut to obtain sensory deprivation. It may be that permanent inhibition results in this case, from connections which are made, but not used, compared with ones which are made late. The second set of studies are by Bentley and Hoy (1970) and Kutsch (1971) on the development of adult motor patterns of cricket flight and song. They used implanted leads to study the two motor neural patterns (as myograms). Flight was elicited by loss of tarsal contact while song was caused by making heat lesions in selected areas of the brains of males. Sixth instar nymphs were capable of generating flight patterns, but these were never maintained as they are in adults four instars later. There must therefore be some final anatomical or physiological addition to the system at the last instar. Song patterns of calling, courtship, and aggression of perfect adult form could be produced only in nymphs in the last instar. These nymphs never sing, but the experiments proved that the neural machinery has been developed and must await the onset of sexual maturity for adequate initiation or release from inhibition. The authors suggested that premature activation of sequentially developed circuits is suppressed by descending inhibition from the brain until maturity.

At the level of tissue culture, there have recently been two instances of marked progress. In cultures of 16-day-old cockroach embryos, intimate relations were established between nerve fibers and myocytes (Aloe and Levi-Montalcini, 1972). In comparable *Drosophila* cultures, junctions were proven to be functional (Seecof et al., 1972) by stimulating the axons and observing the newly formed myocytes contract. This is the first time for any in vitro system that complete differention of neurons, myocytes, and junctions has been obtained.

Genetics and insect neuroethology

There is a rich variety of behavior in many insect species, some of which may be subjected to genetic selection procedures. In *Drosophila*, pioneering work by Hirsch and Boudreau (1958) on the heritability of phototaxis and of Manning (1963) on mating behavior has led to a clear realization that genes influence behavior in highly discrete ways. Benzer (1971) recently listed 26 behavioral mutants of *Drosophila* in six categories, though each of these affects the manner in which the fly behaves rather than affecting Lorenzian "units" of behavioral sequence, which include uncoordinated, nonclimbing, arrhythmic, nonoptomotor reactions. That behavioral units are subject to Mendelian laws has also been shown for certain strains of bees by Rothenbuhler (1964a, b). The bees, termed *hygienic*, normally remove dead larval honey bees from the comb. There are two subunits of the behavior: uncapping and removal of dead larvae. When crossed with a strain not showing this behavior, termed *unhygienic*, the progeny are all unhygienic. But a backcross of the hybrids to the recessive, hygienic strain leads to a simple segregation into four equal groups: (1) bees that uncap only and do not remove dead corpses; (2) bees that do not uncap but remove dead larvae if the cap is first removed by the investigator; (3) ones that do both, i.e., are hygienic; (4) ones that do neither, i.e., are unhygienic. These investigations clearly demonstrate genetic control not just of postural and taxic nervous mechanisms, but of meaningful bits of a complex behavior sequence having several components.

A few of the *Drosophila* mutants have been subjected to preliminary neurophysiological analysis, representing technical feats in view of the size of the fly. Excellent electroretinograms of eyes of the nonphototaxic forms were obtained and found to be markedly different from those of normal eyes (Hotta and Benzer, 1969). Hyperkinetic male mutants are distinguished by showing a specific rhythmic leg shaking during etherization and Ikeda and Kaplan (1970a, b) have shown that these movements are initiated by thoracic neurons. They recorded intracellularly from an unidentified neuron 50 mV action potentials associated with the rhythm.

Unfortunately, since *Drosophila* is so small, progress at the cellular level is not likely to be advanced very far. Of more promise as an experimental animal is the cricket, which is large enough for insertion of two or three electrodes at a time into identified cells. The generation time of some tropical species at 35°C is a mere six weeks! Bentley (1971) took advantage of different numbers of pulses in a trill within a call in the calling song of wild-type *Teleogryllus oceanicus* compared with those occurring in the closely related *T. commodus*. The two species can be mated, and although the F_1 females are sterile, the F_1 males are fertile and can be backcrossed to either parent type. Since male crickets lack a Y chromosome, genes located on the X chromosome received from the maternal parent are unduplicated, and phenotypic differences in the songs of the males can be attributed to X chromosomes. Bentley obtained a series of six types of males from wild-type *T. oceanicus* (A), which has the smallest number of pulses, to wild-type *T. commodus* (F), which has the most. A single motor nerve impulse can determine a pulse, and the number in a trill in the range studied was 2, 3, 4, 5, 6 or 2 × 7 (Figure 5). Hence he could make the important deduction that "genetically derived information

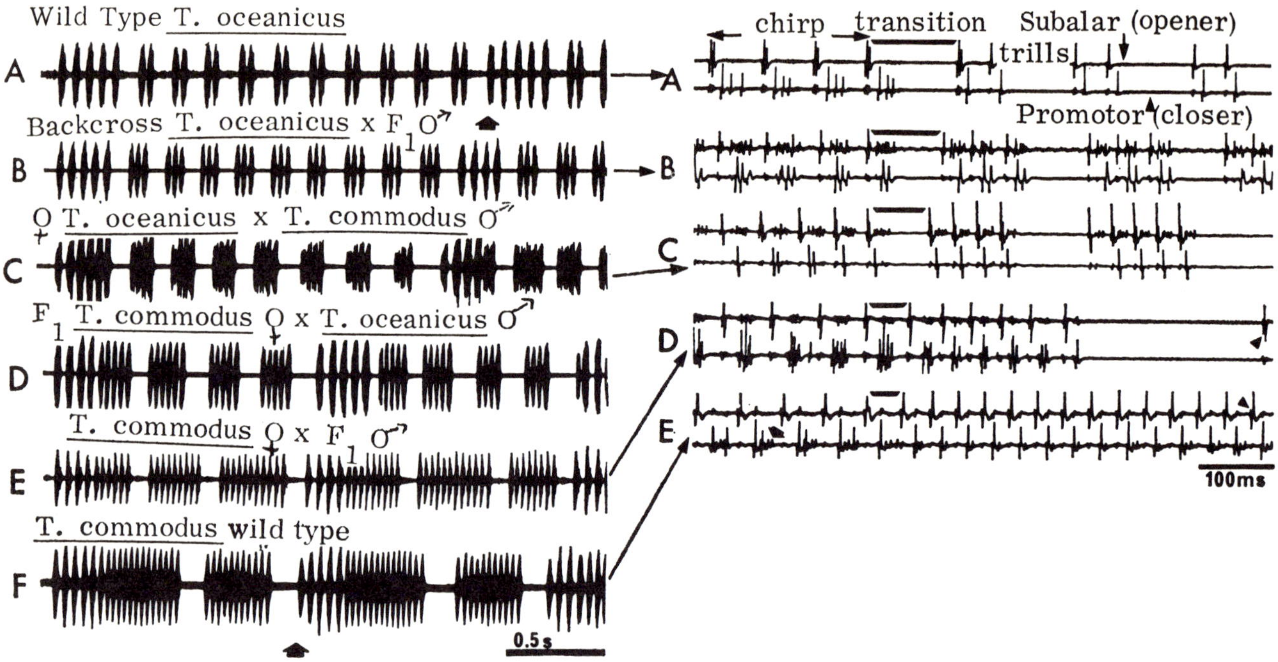

FIGURE 5 Genetics and physiology of sound production by male tropical crickets of the genus *Teleogryllus*. The calling song starts with a single chirp containing 4 to 6 pulses, followed after a transition by several trills. The species *T. oceanicus* has 2 pulses per trill whilst another species *T. commodus* has 14. F_1 males of the species cross are fertile and were backcrossed to parent types yielding a series with varying extents of parental characteristics. The series, presented above, resulted in trills containing 3 (B), 4 (C), 5 (D), and 6 (E) pulses. At left are shown sound patterns at a slow time base speed, while at right are shown electromyograms from a wing opener (*upper*: subalar) and a closer (*lower*: promotor) muscle unit on a faster time base. From Bentley (1971).

is adequate to specify the difference of a single impulse in the output of homologous neurons from different genotypes."

Central versus peripheral control

As investigators began to think about neural mechanisms underlying behavior, old controversies came to the foreground, the most compelling of which was whether or not the Pavlovian mechanistic view, "behavior is reflexes," is acceptable. In the thirties, the emerging ethologists, especially Lorenz (review, 1950) and Tinbergen (review, 1951), guided in part by von Holst, were finding that many acts of behavior appear long after a stimulus has ceased or, in many instances, in the complete absence of an external stimulus. Hess (1943) and von Holst and von St. Paul (1963) found centers in vertebrate brain stems that caused discrete, easily recognized complex behavioral acts to occur when electrically stimulated, whatever the environment. In invertebrates Wells (1950) found intrinsic rhythms related to feeding and defecation cycles in small pieces of isolated tissue of lugworms, and Huber (1962) evoked locomotor and song patterns in crickets by local brain lesions. With a lucky lesion, a male cricket will sing continually for more than 12 hr. Such experiences shattered forever simplistic behaviorist theories and led to searches to test whether given acts of behavior are endogenously generated or peripherally determined. Wilson (review, 1968) firmly established that the flight pattern of locusts does not require peripheral feedback, and Huber and his associates (e.g. Kutsch and Huber, 1970) have determined that cricket singing is likewise endogenous. The most subtle, complex behavior yet studied in this manner is the courtship by the males of the small grasshopper *Gomphocerippus rufus*, in which elegant experiments have shown it to be largely determined by an endogenous program (Loher and Huber, 1966; Elsner, 1969; Huber and Elsner, 1969).

Now there is increasing agreement that in many behaviors there is a basic central nervous program that only needs to be "turned on" in order to ensure the emergence of a behavioral sequence. Correct performance of the relevant movements nevertheless requires proprioceptive feedback for control of the details of the motor impulse patterns.

WALKING The classical view was that walking consists of a series of resistance reflexes, with coordination between legs both within one half of the ganglion and across it. Following an amputation, insects switch very rapidly to a new appropriate gait, a fact that hardly seemed compatible with a central rhythm. Yet Wilson (1966) showed that the changes are not really highly complex and are compatible with control from a rather simple basic central program. When Pearson (1972) removed all sensory input from leg receptors in cockroach preparations, he still obtained reciprocal output in antagonistic leg motorneurons (Figure 1C). This observation does not prove the central program hypothesis but clearly shows that at least part of the necessary neuronal machinery is present entirely within the central nervous system.

Delcomyn (1971a, b) analyzed limb movements from high-speed motion picture film, both of normal and amputated cockroaches. He concluded from the observations that while there may be a central basic program, proprioceptive feedback is undoubtedly of great importance. Later, in a computer-aided electrophysiological study in which legs were forced to move sinusoidally (Delcomyn, 1971c), he found that the intraleg reflexes are such as to augment leg thrust. This is of considerable general interest, because several independent studies on crustaceans (e.g., MacMillan and Dando, 1973) have come to a similar conclusion. Thus it seems that there is a central inherent program that directs locomotory movements but that its output alone tends to evoke weak movements in some systems. In these systems, motor outputs are enhanced by positive feedback during movements. In the cockroach, the program's output is already approximately correctly phased for all legs, including alternating excitation of antagonists.

There are indications of a comparable situation in some mammalian behavior. For example, facial grooming in mice occurs in a basically normal manner following deafferentation, even in the muscles of the stumps of amputated forelegs (Fentress, 1972).

It might be expected that sometimes in a generally excited preparation, a spontaneous turning on of one of the program generators, especially that for walking, would occur. If this happened at a time when an intracellular electrode was placed in a motorneuron or interneuron, one might get clues as to the mechanism involved. Most of the common movement patterns that insects make, such as respiration, walking, song, and other courtship and sexual movements, involve rhythmical repetitions of contractions. Accordingly, a major part of the endogenous neural machinery is often considered to consist of one or more "oscillators" (Wilson, 1967; Davis, 1969; Davis and Kennedy, 1972a, b). A specific search for a central flight oscillator in the locust failed to find one (Page, 1970). But interesting oscillatory membrane potential swings of large size occurring at the relevant natural rhythm have now been observed intracellularly in three situations: sound production, flight, and walking rhythm of crickets and locusts (Figure 6). Action potentials in the motor axon of the relevant neurons were monitored by recording extracellularly from the muscle innervated. In all cases there has been a peripheral spike only if the depolarization recorded in the soma reached a critical value. If the soma potential was both large and steeply rising, a close pair, triplet, or quadruplet of impulses was produced. It is thus probable that the wave of depolarization is an electrotonically conducted correlate of the neuropilar dendrite/neurite potential that generates the

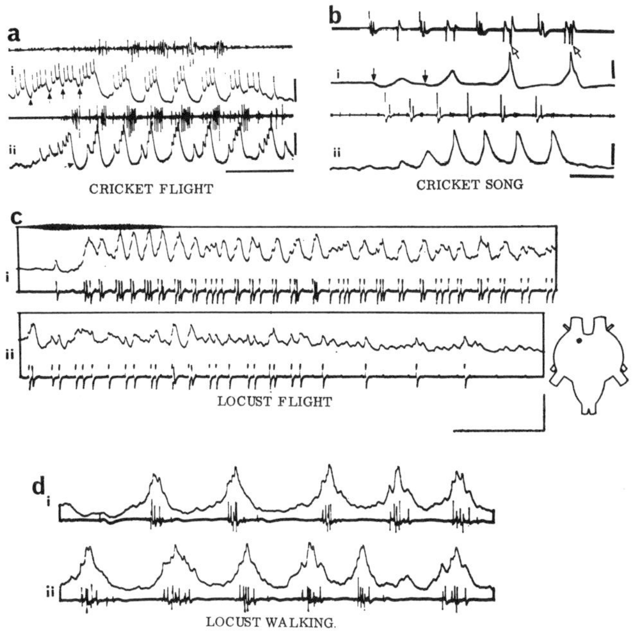

FIGURE 6 Rhythmic membrane potentials occurring in ganglion cells recorded intracellularly. (a) i and ii: Two sequences from cricket during flight patterns—possibly from wing elevator neurons, on lower traces. Extracellular electromyograms from subalar muscles on upper traces. Arrows indicate possible inhibitory activity at start of depressor bursts that drive the subalar muscles. Calibration: vertical, 10 mV; horizontal, 100 msec. From Bentley (1969a). (b) From cricket during singing. Records from unknown wing closers with an intracellular electrode (lower traces) and extracellular from motor nerves (upper traces). Filled arrows: onset of polarizing activity; open arrows: efferent impulses following ganglion cell spikes. Calibration: vertical, 10 mV; horizontal, (i) 25 msec; (ii) 50 msec. From Bentley (1969b). (c) i and ii: Activity in locust metathoracic flight motorneuron whose location is indicated in the insert, during flight pattern. Activity excited by an air puff applied to the head (monitored via microphone on upper beam). Lower beam: myogram from subalar muscles. Note exact correspondence with spikes on intracellular record. The entire sequence takes place during a plateau of depolarization that is maintained during the flight sequence but gradually subsides towards termination. Calibration: 10 mV; 250 msec. From Hoyle and Burrows (1973b). (d) i and ii: Continuous records from locust posterior fast flexor during spontaneously occurring flexions of the tibia. Electromyogram (upper trace) is from femur and shows that reciprocal extensor activity was very weak. Calibration: 10 mV; 500 msec. From Hoyle and Burrows (1973b).

spikes. The nature of the waves is at the present time uncertain. Either they are due to many small, summating EPSPs, to an electrotonically coupled oscillator neuron (Mendelson, 1971), or they are intrinsically generated in the neuropilar segment of the motorneuron itself.

Some spontaneously occurring potential swings of about 15 mV peak-to-peak causing output in flexor tibiae motorneurons recorded by Hoyle and Burrows (1973b) had a frequency of about 2 Hz, characteristic of locust stepping during walking. But in these cases the antagonistic slow extensor motorneuron (the fast extensor fires only in jumping) was silent and the leg moved hardly at all. In this case therefore, the action closely resembled what might be expected from a spontaneously firing "oscillator." The membrane potential swings in the flight motorneurons were more than 10 mV peak-to-peak in the soma and occurred at the flight rhythm of 19 Hz.

Neuronal circuitry

JUMP RESPONSE The simple grasshopper and locust escape behavior, jumping, is the one in which most progress is being made toward a reasonably complete analysis of underlying neuronal events. All the motorneurons involved, six flexors and the single fast extensor, have been located and examined intracellularly during elicitation of the reflex (Hoyle and Burrows, 1973a). Three interneurons associated with flexion have been located and recorded from, and the action of some others can be inferred.

In a jump response the left and right fast extensors fire simultaneously and at similar rates; this coordination is not achieved by direct excitatory connections between them but by independent simultaneous activation (Hoyle and Burrows, 1973a). This requires input from chordotonal organs located in the femora (Bassler, 1968) that are stimulated by the rapid strong flexion of the tibia, which is always the initial action in a jump response and is due to a fast flexor neuron. The next stage is a simultaneous inhibitory input to the flexor motorneurons and an excitatory one to the fast extensor motorneurons, of both sides. Once an action potential has been fired by the fast extensor it re-excites itself. As judged by the delay and number of summating, facilitating EPSPs involved, this is probably via collaterals and interneurons. The net result is that if the general excitatory level is high, as it usually is after stimuli of the kind that cause jumps, the two FETi fire bursts of impulses that fully tetanize the extensor muscles, causing take-off. The jump is completed by a flexion of the tibia. This is achieved in part by delayed excitation occurring automatically via an interneuron that synapses with the flexors and is excited by a fast extensor collateral.

Earlier stages in the initiation of the jump response are obscure. It has been assumed for many years that the response, like the startle response of the cockroach, is due to action of giant fibers (Roeder, 1948; Cook, 1951). But recently, the giant fibers were shown to be unnecessary in the cockroach (Parnas and Dagan, 1971); their function may be simply to arrest other ongoing activity preparatory to execution of the escape reponse.

In the locust the only neurons so far discovered that have axons to both sides of the ganglion, which could therefore mediate a bilateral response, are the central dorsal giants (Crossman et al., 1971). These do always fire prior to the jump response (Dagan and Hoyle, unpublished), but their behavioral role is not yet known.

COMMAND FIBERS Hughes and Wiersma (1960) discovcovered interneurons in crayfish circumesophagel connectives that cause patterned, relatively complex movements to occur when stimulated by a simple train. The movements of some parts, for example the swimmerets, are rhythmical, continuing ones. Wiersma and Ikeda (1964) termed such fibers "command" fibers. Fibers that have some aspects in common with these have been found in only one insect thus far (Figure 7), a small grasshopper *Gastrimargus africanus* by Elsner (1969). The responses he obtained were rhythmical up and down leg movements.

The actual functional role of such fibers in the insect has not been established. It may be that these fibers are no more than general excitatory interneurons (Hoyle, 1964)

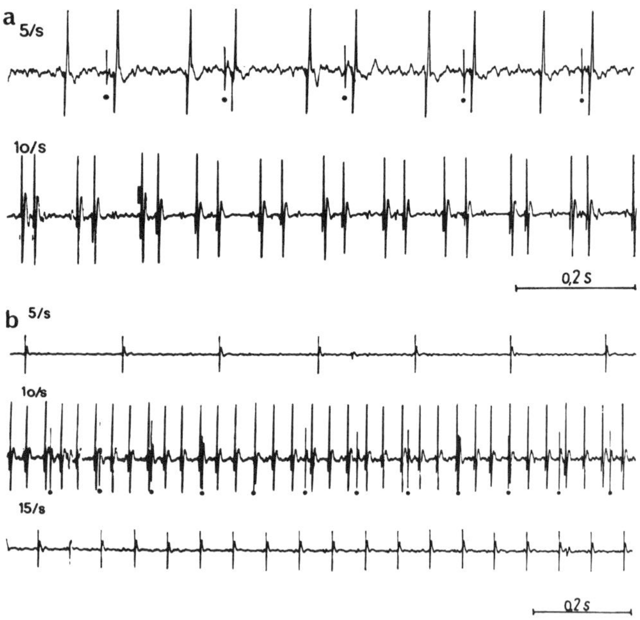

FIGURE 7 Rhythmical muscle activity not related 1:1 to stimulus elicited in a grasshopper (*Gastrimargus africanus*) by stimulation of axon bundles in cervical connectives. (a) Paired outputs for single inputs. (b) Sequences of bursts at fixed long intervals elicited only at 10 Hz not at 5 or 15 Hz. From Elsner (1969).

that cause autogenic circuits to come into operation. If a brain is shown to really use these fibers to "command" the lower motor centers to "do their thing" by issuing continuing trains, that will be a major step in our understanding of neuroethology.

Excitation of Antagonists The traditional, Sherringtonian view of the use of antagonists as simple reciprocators during movements has generally been accepted as the norm for operation in insect movements, although Hoyle (1964) found that in long-term recordings from freely walking locusts the electrical records suggested a high degree of cocontraction. The problem was easily resolvable with the aid of two microelectrodes placed in somas of antagonistic pairs of motorneurons because the activity in the somas cannot be misinterpreted. The data for several pairs of antagonists all showed clearly that the synaptic excitation causing movements would lead to cocontraction in at least 20% of the cases. About 50% of inputs are of simple reciprocal nature and in the remainder co-excitation and reciprocal excitation are mixed (Figure 8).

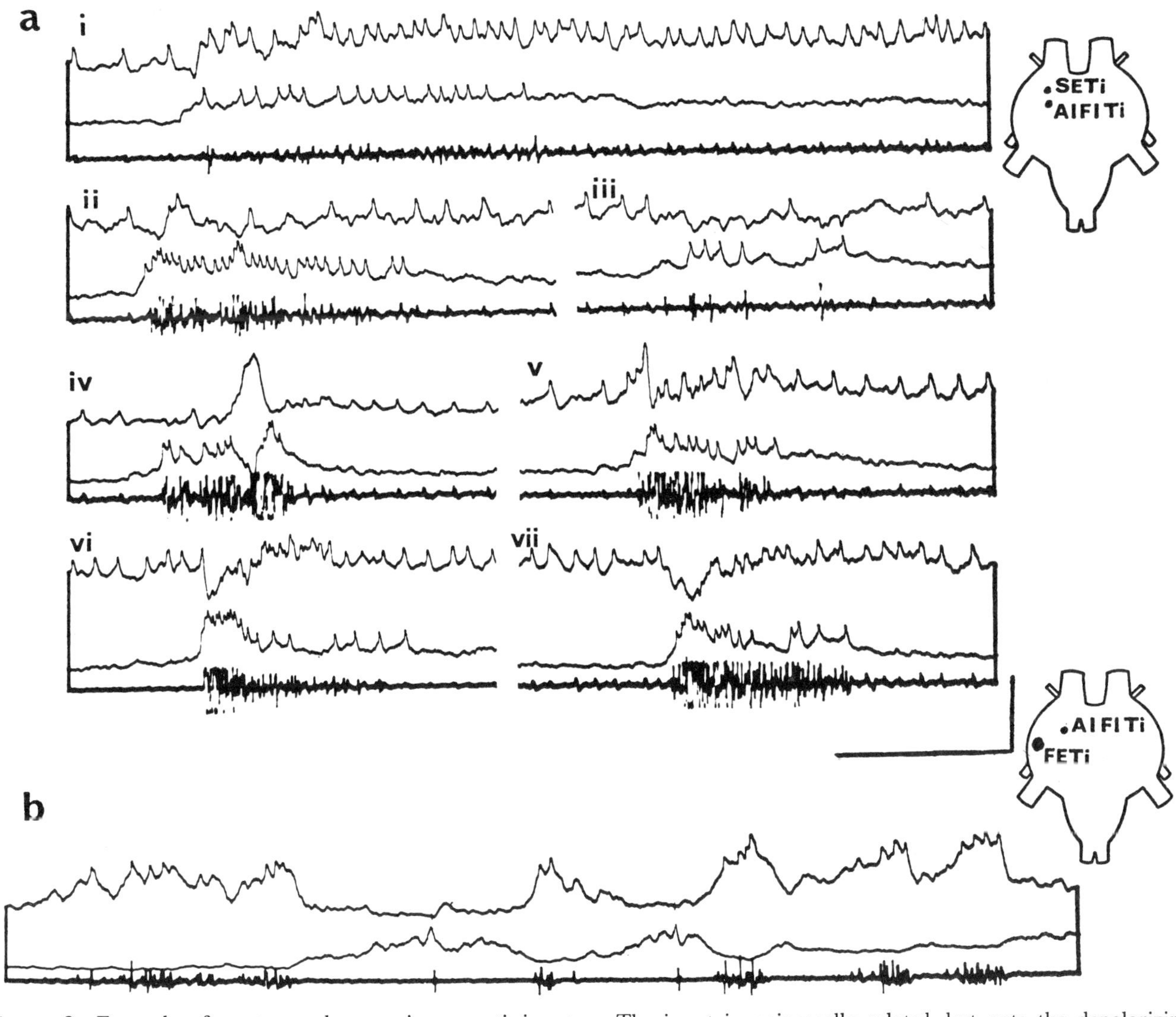

Figure 8 Examples of spontaneously occurring synaptic input to antagonists of the locust metathoracic ganglion during simultaneous intracellular recordings. (a) Slow extensor tibiae (upper traces) and anterior intermediate flexor (middle traces). Note that the slow extensor may be excited either: at the same time as the flexor leading to cocontraction [(a) i and (a) ii]; completely reciprocally [(a) iii and (a) vii]; or mixed coactivation and reciprocal activation [(a) ii and (a) vi]. (b) Fast extensor tibiae (upper traces) and anterior intermediate flexor (middle traces). The input is reciprocally related, but note the depolarizing response in the flexor following firing of the extensor. The locations of the neuron somas from which the intracellular recordings were made are shown in the two insert diagrams of the metathoracic ganglion from the ventral aspect. The lower traces denote extracellular electromyograms recorded with wires placed in the femur. Calibration: 10 mV; 250 msec. From Hoyle and Burrows (1973a).

Entrainment of Identified Neurons Horridge (1962) found that it is easy to train headless cockroaches and locusts to hold up a leg in order to avoid receiving a shock. Hoyle (1965) made a successful attempt in the locust to train a tonically firing, postural motorneuron to alter its firing rate (Figure 9). The preparation is promising, because it offers the possibility of examining the cellular basis of a learning process. The relevant neuron, the anterior coxal adductor, was localized in the ganglion by Hoyle and Burrows (1973a). A computer program has now been developed that permits automatic entrainment. The discharge of the neuron is stored by a computer that sorts succeeding impulses into a series of bins of spike intervals. By preset instructions, the computer recognises the appearance in the discharge of any significant trend toward consecutive long intervals (equal to a low firing rate). In the whole insect, these would be followed by loss of muscle tone and lowering of the leg. The computer then triggers a stimulator that delivers a shock to a sensory nerve having indirect input to the motorneuron. The result of a few minutes of such training, in which only 5 to 10 shocks are received, is often a stable shift in the interval histogram toward shorter intervals. Examples of before- and after-training histograms photographed directly from the scope face of a Linc-8 computer are given in Figure 9.

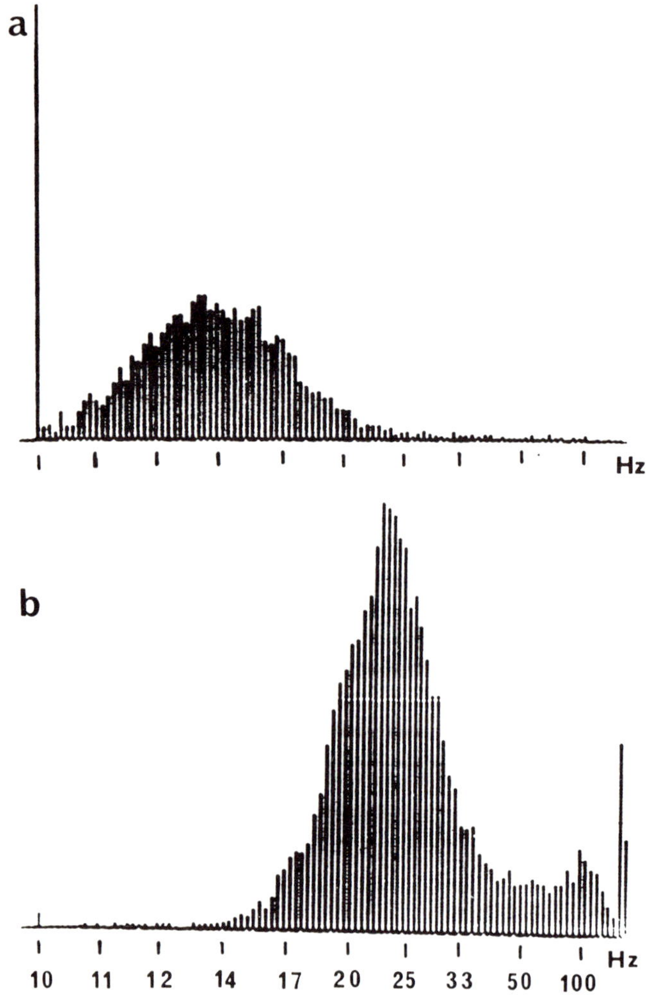

Figure 9 Entrainment of an identified neuron. Computer histogram (on oscilloscope) of discharge of single excitatory axon to anterior coxal adductor. (a) Fresh insect before training. (b) Same insect after applying training program. A weak electric shock was applied to the leg each time successive long intervals, which were accumulated in a single bin, left-hand side of record in (a), had occurred. The preparation responds by stable increased mean firing rate, with almost total lack of long intervals. Records made for equal times, hence more intervals stored in (b). From Tosney and Hoyle (in preparation).

Summary

Among all animals, insects with complex, varied behavior yet small total numbers of nerve cells and very short generation times offer the greatest opportunities for in-depth studies of neural circuits and the ways in which behavior is controlled. Simple electromyograms and nerve impulse recordings are easily obtained from freely moving intact animals, providing quantitative information about the motor output. Recently developed techniques have enabled intracellular recordings to be made from nerve cell bodies in the ganglia, in preparations in which there is at least limited behavior. The recordings are followed by dye injections that in turn permit both neuron localization and the following of dendritic and axonal pathways. Preliminary work on neural integration in locusts is described as well as experiments in which the frequency of firing of a tonic, postural motorneuron is modified by operant conditioning. Work under way in other laboratories on the genetics of insect behavior can be linked to possible underlying neural mechanisms. Developmental and tissue culture studies on cockroach ganglia seem likely to provide basic knowledge on neuronal specificity and the making of functional contacts between neurons.

acknowledgments The original research referred to in this article was supported by National Science Foundation Research Grant No. 32018.

I would like to acknowledge the technical assistance of Lee H. Vernon, Harrison Howard, Betty Moberley, and Julie Pohl, to praise the superb technical skills of my collaborators Dr. Malcolm Burrows and Dr. Dani Dagan, and to commend all fellow workers in the field, especially Dr. David Bentley, Dr. Franz Huber, Dr. Keir Pearson, and Dr. Norbert Elsner.

REFERENCES

ALBRECHT, F. O., 1953. *The Anatomy of the Migratory Locust.* London: Athlone Press.

ALOE, L., and R. LEVI-MONTALCINI, 1972. Interrelation and dynamic activity of visceral muscle and nerve cells from insect embryos in long-term culture. *J. Neurobiol.* 3:3–23.

BASSLER, U., 1968. Zur Steuerung des Springens bei der Wanderheuschrecke *Schistocerca gregaria. Kybernetik* 4:112.

BENTLEY, D. R., 1969a. Intracellular activity in cricket neurons during the generation of behaviour patterns. *J. Insect Physiol.* 15:677–699.

BENTLEY, D. R., 1969b. Intracellular activity in cricket neurons during generation of song patterns. *Z. Vergl. Physiol.* 62:267–283.

BENTLEY, D. R., 1970. A topological map of the locust flight system motor neurons. *J. Insect Physiol.* 16:905–918.

BENTLEY, D. R., 1971. Genetic control of an insect neuronal network. *Science* 174:1139–1141.

BENTLEY, D. R., and R. R. HOY, 1970. Postembryonic development of adult motor patterns in crickets: a neural analysis. *Science* 170:1409–1411.

BENZER, S., 1971. From gene to behavior. *J. Amer. Med. Ass.* 218:1015–1022.

BURROWS, M., and G. HOYLE, 1973. Neural mechanisms underlying behavior in the locust *Schistocerca gregaria.* 3. Topography of limb motorneurons in metathoracic ganglia. *J. Neurobiol.* 4:167–186.

COOK, P. M., 1951. Observations on giant fibers of the nervous system of *Locusta migratoria. Quart. J. Mic. Sci.* 92:297–305.

CROSSMAN, A. R., G. A. KERKUT, R. M. PITMAN, and R. J. WALKER, 1971. Electrically excitable nerve cell bodies in the central ganglia of two insect species *Periplaneta americana* and *Schistocerca gregaria.* Investigation of cell geometry and morphology by intracellular dye injection. *Comp. Biochem. Physiol.* 40(A):579–594.

DAVIS, W. J., 1969. The neural control of swimmeret beating in the lobster. *J. Exp. Biol.* 50:99–117.

DAVIS, W. J., and D. KENNEDY, 1972a. Command interneurons controlling swimmeret movements in the lobster. I. Types of effects on motorneurons. *J. Neurophysiol.* 35:1–12.

DAVIS, W. J., and D. KENNEDY, 1972b. Command interneurons controlling swimmeret movements in the lobster. II. Interaction of effects on motorneurons. *J. Neurophysiol.* 35:13–19.

DELCOMYN, F., 1971a. The locomotion of the cockroach *Periplaneta americana. J. Exp. Biol.* 54:443–452.

DELCOMYN, F., 1971b. The effect of limb amputation on locomotion in the cockroach *Periplaneta americana. J. Exp. Biol.* 54:453–469.

DELCOMYN, F., 1971c. Computer aided analysis of a locomotor leg reflex in the cockroach *Periplaneta americana. Z. Vergl. Physiol.* 74:427–445.

EDWARDS, J. S., 1969. Postembryonic development and regeneration of the insect nervous system. *Adv. Ins. Physiol.* 6:97–137.

EDWARDS, J. S., and J. PALKA, 1971. Neural regeneration: delayed formation of central contacts by insect sensory cells. *Science* 172:591–594.

EDWARDS, J. S., and T. S. SAHOTA, 1967. Regeneration of a sensory system: the formation of central connections by normal and transplanted cerci of the house cricket *Acheta domesticus. J. Exp. Zool.* 166:387–396.

ELSNER, N., 1968. Die neuromuskularen Grundlagen des Werbeverhaltens der roten Keulenheuschrecke *Gomphocerippurufus* (L.). *Z. Vergl. Physiol.* 60:308–350.

ELSNER, N., 1969. Kommandofasern im Zentralnervensystem der Heuschrecke *Gastrimargus africanus* (Oedipodinae). *Verh. Deutsch. Ges. Zool.* 33:465–471.

ELSNER, N., 1973. The central nervous control of courtship behavior in the grasshopper *Gomphocerippus rufus* (L.) (Orthoptera: Acrididae). 1971. *Sympos. Invert. Neurobiol.*

FENTRESS, J., 1972. Development of patterning of movement sequences in inbred mice. In *The Biology of Behavior*, J. Kiger, ed. Eugene, Oregon: Oregon State University Press.

HAGIWARA, S., and A. WATANABE, 1956. Discharges in motorneurons of cicada. *J. Cell. Comp. Physiol.* 47:415–428.

HESS, W. R., 1943. Das Zwischenhirn als Koordinationsorgan. *Helv. Physiol. Pharmacol. Acta* 1:549–565.

HIRSCH, J., and J. C. BOUDREAU, 1958. Studies in experimental behavior genetics. 1. The heritability of phototaxis in a population of *Drosophila melanogaster. J. Comp. Physiol. Psychol.* 51:647–651.

HORRIDGE, G. A., 1962. Learning leg position by the ventral nerve cord in headless insects. *Proc. Roy. Soc.* [*Biol.*] 157:33–52.

HOTTA, Y., and S. BENZER, 1969. Abnormal electroretinograms in visual mutants of *Drosophila. Nature* (*London*) 222:354–365.

HOYLE, G. 1953. Potassium ions and insect nerve muscle. *J. Exp. Biol.* 30:121–135.

HOYLE, G., 1957. Nervous control of insect muscles. In *Recent Advances in Invertebrate Physiology.* Eugene, Oregon: University of Oregon Publications, pp. 73–98.

HOYLE, G., 1964. Exploration of neuronal mechanisms underlying behavior of insects. In *Neural Theory and Modeling*, R. Reiss, ed. Stanford, Calif.: Stanford University Press, pp. 346–376.

HOYLE, G., 1965. Neurophysiological studies on "learning" in headless insects. In *The Physiology of the Insect Central Nervous System*, J. E. Treherne, and J. W. L. Beament, eds. London and New York: Academic Press, pp. 203–232.

HOYLE, G., and M. BURROWS, 1970. Intracellular studies on identified neurons of insects. *Fed. Proc.* 29:1920A.

HOYLE, G., and M. BURROWS, 1973a. Neural mechanisms underlying behavior in the locust *Schistocerca gregaria.* 1. Physiology of identified neurons in the metathoracic ganglion. *J. Neurobiol.* 4:3–41.

HOYLE, G., and M. BURROWS, 1973b. Neural mechanisms underlying behavior in the locust *Schistocerca gregaria.* 2. Integrative activity in metathoracic neurons. *J. Neurobiol.* 4:43–67.

HUBER, F. 1962. Central nervous control of sound production in crickets and some speculation on its evolution. *Evol.* 16:429–442.

HUBER, F., 1971. Nervose Grundlagen der akustiscken Kommunikation bei Insekten. *Acad. Wiss. Phein-West.* 205:41–84.

HUBER, F., and N. ELSNER, 1969. Die Organisation des Werbegesanges der Heuschrecke *Gomphocerippus rufus* L. in Abhangigkeit von zentralen und peripheren Bedingungen. *Z. Vergl. Physiol.* 65:389–443.

HUGHES, G. M., and C. A. G. WIERSMA, 1960. The co-ordination of swimmeret movements in the crayfish *Procambarus clarkii* (Girard). *J. Exp. Biol.* 37:657–670.

IKEDA, K., and W. D. KAPLAN, 1970a. Patterned neural activity of a mutant *Drosophila melanogaster. Proc. Nat. Acad. Sci.* (*USA*) 66:765–772.

IKEDA, K., and W. D. KAPLAN, 1970b. Unilaterally patterned

neural activity of gynandromorphs, mosaic for a neurological mutant of *Drosophila melanogaster. Proc. Nat. Acad. Sci.* (*USA*) 67:1480–1487.

Kerkut, G. A., R. M. Pitman, and R. J. Walker, 1968. Electrical activity in insect nerve cell bodies. *Life Sci.* 7:605–607.

Kerkut, G. A., R. M. Pitman, and R. J. Walker, 1969. Sensitivity of neurons of the insect central nervous system to iontophoretically applied acetylcholine or GABA. *Nature* (*London*) 222:1075–1076.

Kutsch, W., 1971. The development of the flight pattern in the desert locust *Schistocerca gregaria. Z. Vergl. Physiol.* 74:156–168.

Kutsch, W., and F. Huber, 1970. Zentrale versus periphere Kontrolle des Gesanges von Grillen (*Gryllus campestris*). *Z. Vergl. Physiol.* 67:140–159.

Loher, W., and F. Huber, 1966. Nervous and endocrine control of behavior in a grasshopper (*Gomphocerippus rufus* L. Acrididae). *Sympos. Soc. Exp. Biol.* 20:381–400.

Lorenz, K. Z., 1950. The comparative method in studying innate behavior patterns. *Sympos. Soc. Exp. Biol.* 4:221–268.

MacMillan, D. L., and M. R. Dando, 1973. Tension receptors associated with the apodemes of muscles in the walking legs of the crab *Cancer magister.* In *Marine Biology and Behavior* (in press).

Manning, A., 1963. Selection for mating speed in *Drosophila melanogaster* based on the behavior of one sex. *Anim. Behav.* 11:116–120.

Maynard, D. M., 1956. Electrical activity in the cockroach cerebrum. *Nature* (*London*) 177:529–530.

Mendelson, M., 1971. Oscillator neurons in crustacean ganglia. *Science* 171:1170–1173.

Narahashi, T., 1965. The physiology of insect axons. In *The Physiology of the Insect Central Nervous System*, J. E. Treherne, and J. W. L. Beament, eds. London and New York: Academic Press, pp. 1–20.

Page, C. H., 1970. Unit responses in the metathoracic ganglion of the flying locust. *Comp. Biochem. Physiol.* 37:565–571.

Parnas, I., and D. Dagan, 1971. Functional organizations of giant axons in the central nervous systems of insects. New aspects. *Adv. Insect Physiol.* 8:95–143.

Pearson, K. G., 1972. Central programming and reflex control of walking in the cockroach. *J. Exp. Biol.* 56:173–193.

Roeder, K. D., 1948. Organization of the ascending giant fiber system in the cockroach (*Periplaneta americana*). *J. Exp. Zool.* 108:243–262.

Rothenbuhler, W. C., 1964a. Behavior genetics of nest cleaning in honey-bees. 1. Responses of four inbred lines to disease-killed brood. *Anim. Behav.* 12:578–583.

Rothenbuhler, W. C., 1964b. Behavior genetics of nest cleaning in honey-bees. 4. Responses of F_1 and back-cross generations to disease-killed brood. *Amer. Zool.* 4:111–123.

Rowe, E. C., 1960. Activity of single nerve cells in an insect thoracic ganglion. *Anat. Rec.* 137:389 (Abstract).

Rowe, E. C., 1969. Microelectrode records from a cockroach thoracic ganglion: Synaptic potentials and temporal patterns of spike activity. *Comp. Biochem. Physiol.* 30:529–539.

Runion, H. I., and P. N. R. Usherwood, 1966. A new approach to neuromuscular analysis in the intact free-walking insect preparation. *J. Insect Physiol.* 12:1255–1263.

Seecof, R. L., R. L. Teplitz, I. Gerson, K. Ikeda, and J. J. Donady, 1972. Differentiation of neuromuscular junctions in cultures of embryonic *Drosophila* cells. *Proc. Nat. Acad. Sci.* (*USA*) 69: 566–570.

Sperry, R. W., 1943. Effect of 180 degree rotation of the retinal field on visuomotor co-ordination. *J. Exp. Zool.* 92:263–279.

Spira, M. E., I. Parnas, and F. Bergmann, 1969. Histological and electrophysiological studies on the giant axons of the cockroach *Periplaneta americana. J. Exp. Biol.* 50:629–634.

Stretton, A. O. W., and E. A. Kravitz, 1968. Neuronal geometry: Determination with a technique of intracellular dye injection. *Science* 162:132–134.

Tinbergen, N., 1951. *The Study of Instinct.* London: Oxford University Press.

Usherwood, P. N. R., and H. I. Runion, 1970. Analysis of the mechanical responses of metathoracic extensor tibiae muscles of free-walking locusts. *J. Exp. Biol.* 52:39–58.

von Holst, E., and U. von St. Paul, 1963. On the functional organization of drives. *An. Behav.* 11:1–20.

Weiss, P., 1950. Experimental analysis of co-ordination by the disarrangement of central peripheral relations. *Sympos. Soc. Exp. Biol.* 4:92–111.

Wells, G. P., 1950. Spontaneous activity cycles in polychaete worms. *Sympos. Soc. Exp. Biol.* 4:127–142.

Wiersma, C. A. G., 1959. Coding and decoding in the nervous system. *Engineering and Science Monthly* (Calif. Inst. Technol.) 23:21–24.

Wiersma, C. A. G., and K. Ikeda, 1964. Interneurons commanding swimmeret movements in the crayfish *Procambarus clarkii* (Girard). *Comp. Biochem. Physiol.* 12:509–525.

Wiesel, T. N., and D. H. Hubel, 1963. Single-cell responses in striate cortex of kittens deprived of vision in one eye. *J. Neurophysiol.* 26:1003–1017.

Wiesel, T. N., and D. H. Hubel, 1965. Comparison of the effects of unilateral and bilateral eye closure on cortical unit responses in kittens. *J. Neurophysiol.* 28:1029–1040.

Wigglesworth, V. B., 1939. *The Principles of Insect Physiology*, 1st Ed., London: Methuen.

Wilson, D. M., 1966. Insect walking. *Ann. Rev. Entom.* 11:103–122.

Wilson, D. M., 1967. An approach to the problem of control of rhythmic behavior. In *Invertebrate Nervous Systems*, C. A. G. Wiersma, ed. Chicago: Chicago University Press, pp. 219–229.

Wilson, D. M., 1968. The nervous control of insect flight and related behavior. *Adv. Insect Physiol.* 5:289–338.

36 A Comparison of the Visual Behavior of a Predatory Arthropod with That of a Mammal

MICHAEL F. LAND

ABSTRACT Any predator has the tasks of locating prey, identifying it, and capturing it. These operations necessarily involve specializations: On the sensory side for high spatial acuity and on the motor side for speed of action. The chapter is concerned chiefly with the visual system of jumping spiders, which catch flies by stalking them. Each of the four pairs of simple eyes—the fixed side eyes and movable principal eyes—plays a different role in prey capture and courtship, and techniques are described by which the several kinds of control mechanism involved can be separated and examined. Specific examples are the control of turning by the side eyes during the localization of moving stimuli and the part played by scanning movements of the principal eyes in identifying seen stimuli as potential prey or potential mates.

Introduction

To DRAW USEFUL conclusions from a comparison between animals with totally different evolutionary histories, it is necessary to choose species whose life styles are similar. Then it is possible to begin to sort out how much the organization of an animal's behavior reflects the principles of construction of the nervous system peculiar to a phylum and how much is due to convergent evolution caused by similarities in the tasks performed. Predatory animals, especially those that hunt visually, always have interesting behavior that is usually comprehensible to an observer, because the goals of many of the different components are clear. They are thus attractive subjects on which to base a comparative study. There are relatively few terrestrial arthropods that catch active prey by stalking them, in the manner of a mammalian carnivore. There is, however, one group, the jumping spiders (*Salticidae*), that do so; the strategy they adopt in catching flies is sufficiently similar to that of a cat catching a bird—to creep toward the prey undetected until the chance of escape is small, and then spring—that it is worthwhile to enquire further into the optical, neural, and behavioral specializations that make this possible. This chapter is concerned chiefly with examining parallels and contrasts in visually directed behavior; more detailed studies of salticid behavior are given by Drees (1952), Crane (1949), and Heil (1936); of visual anatomy by Land (1969a) and Eakin and Brandenburger (1971); of visual optics by Land (1969a, 1969b) and Homann (1928); and of motor control by Land (1971, 1972).

MICHAEL F. LAND School of Biological Sciences, University of Sussex, Falmer, Sussex, England

Optical organization

All spiders have either 8 or 6 simple eyes, each constructed with a lens that is part of the cuticle, a cellular but transparent *vitreous*, and a retina containing up to 10^4 primary receptors but with no ganglion cells or other neurons in the eye itself. In jumping spiders, 6 of the 8 eyes are particularly well developed and fall into two groups: The fixed lateral eyes (Figure 1) that between them cover a field of view extending the full 360° around the animal, including a 25° region of binocular overlap anteriorly, and the principal eyes with a much longer focal length but very restricted field of view—between 1 and 5° laterally by 20° vertically. However, the retinae of the principal eyes are movable, so that the range of vision of these eyes during movements is extended to approximately 35° on either side of the midline in the horizontal plane, and by a similar amount vertically (Land, 1969b).

The lateral eyes are movement detectors, and there is no behavioral evidence to indicate that they do anything else. When something moves in the visual environment—whether it is an insect, another spider, or even a car on the street—the spider turns to face it, and this turn is mediated by the lateral eyes. In the posterolateral eyes the receptor spacing is everywhere between 1 and 1.5°, and any object that subtends at least this angle and moves through a similar angle (i.e., from one receptor to the next) stands an equal chance of evoking a turn (Land, 1971). In the anterolateral eyes the situation is similar, except that, in

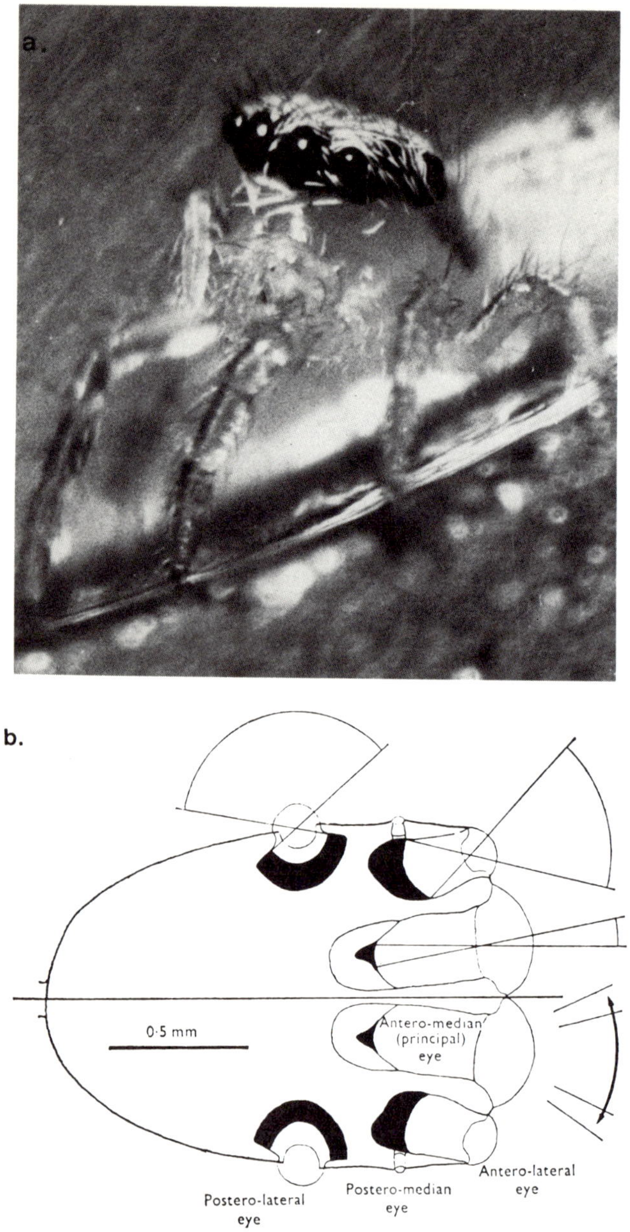

FIGURE 1 (a) Juvenile jumping spider (*Metaphidippus harfordi*: 2 mm long) showing the eyes on the prosoma. (b) Diagrammatic longitudinal section through the prosoma of a jumping spider, showing the fields of view of the eyes in the horizontal plane. For the right principal eye the field is shown as it is extended by lateral eye-movements. In some spiders (e.g., *Salticus*) the fields of the posterolateral eyes meet behind the animal.

the region of the retina close to the spider's axis, the receptor spacing decreases to 30 min, and in this region turns can be evoked by much smaller objects.

By contrast, the principal eyes have much higher resolution and, as Homann (1928) showed by blinding each set of eyes in turn, the principal eyes are concerned with tracking objects that have already been located by the lateral eyes and with pattern recognition. These retinae have a complex structure with 4 layers of receptors, and it is argued elsewhere that this layering is used to compensate for longitudinal chromatic aberration (Land, 1969a) in a manner similar to the layered arrangement of cones in fish retinae (Eberle, 1967); there is now ample behavioral and physiological evidence that jumping spiders possess at least dichromatic color vision. However, of more interest to the present discussion is the finding that the retina is arranged in a *foveal* manner, with receptor separations in the central part of about 10 min increasing in the upper and lower extremities to nearly 45 min. During certain eye movements (see below) this central region of retina is directed to stimuli in the visual field, so that the use of the term fovea is functionally as well as anatomically correct.

In mammals, at least in carnivores and primates including man, the functions of the peripheral and central regions of the retina are quite different, the former being concerned largely with detecting objects to the side and directing the retinal center toward them by a saccadic eye movement, a head movement, or a combination of the two. Tasks requiring higher resolution—pattern recognition and tracking of small objects—are performed by the foveal region. In jumping spiders the same division of labor exists, but the different functions are performed by different eyes. It is interesting that the task of movement detection, which requires relatively low resolution and for which movement of the eye itself is actually a potential source of confusion, is performed here by fixed eyes of short focal length (in *Metaphidippus aeneolus* the focal length of the posterolateral eyes is 174 μm, nearly 3 times shorter than that of the principal eyes which is 512 μm). This optical division of labor results in an enormous economy of space, because a spherical eye built on the vertebrate plan would have to have a long focal length to provide the required resolution at the center and would occupy a volume nearly 3^3 times that of the posterolateral eyes, which provide wide-field coverage. As it is, this space, nearly the entire volume of the spider's prosoma, is saved, and the fovea of the system is confined to a long but narrow tubular eye. It is tempting to argue that the system evolved by jumping spiders is much the more efficient.

Last, because jumping spiders have simple eyes of wide aperture, their resolving power is both theoretically and practically greater than that of their prey with compound eyes. The Rayleigh criterion sets a limit of at best 30 min to the resolution achievable by a compound eye of the apposition type—3 times worse than that of the principal eyes of these spiders (see Barlow, 1952). Ophthalmoscopic examination of the retinae of jumping spiders, which

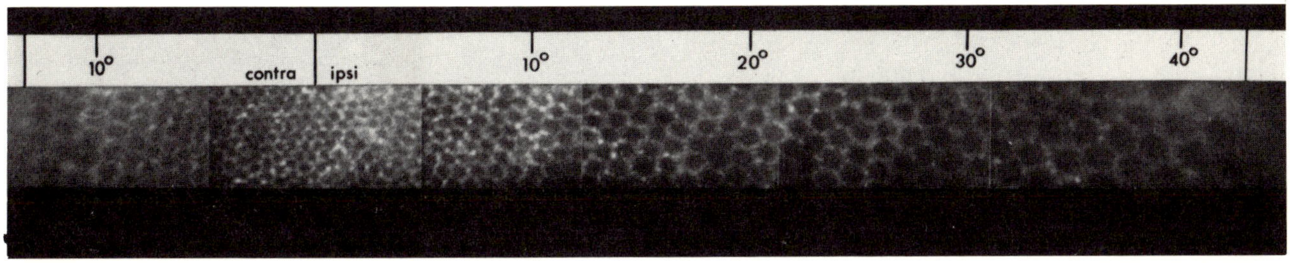

FIGURE 2 Photographic montage of a 5°-wide horizontal strip across the retina of the fixed anterolateral eye of *Salticus scenicus*, taken through the spider's own lens using an ophthalmoscope (Land, 1969b). The field of view of the eye extends from 43° to the ipsilateral side of the body axis to 13° across the axis. The lighter lattice is caused by light scattering from the melanin granules that partition the individual receptors from each other: These are contained in the dark hexagons. In the region of the body axis, the angular separation of individual receptors is 3 times less than at the peripheries: This is not the result of optical distortion.

makes use of, and is therefore limited by, the optical quality of the lens and ocular media, demonstrates convincingly that the eyes are optically excellent and that the limit to resolution is set by receptor density (see Land, 1969a, and Figure 2). The minimum receptor separation of 10 min in the principal retinae is just over one order of magnitude larger than in man but less than in any other invertebrate except the cephalopod molluscs.

Control of movement

Human eye movements have among other tasks the two of locating objects of interest and of tracking their movements. Locating usually involves a saccade, whose control system is *open* in nature in that the size of the movement is determined prior to its execution and is not modified by visual feedback during its progress. Smooth-pursuit eye movements, on the other hand, necessarily involve continuous feedback (see Bizzi and Evarts, 1971). In catching a fly, the spider has the same two tasks—location and tracking—and it is interesting that the two control systems concerned are similar to their mammalian analogues: Turns initiated by the lateral eyes do not require visual feedback for their accurate completion, whereas the small turns used in tracking, for which the principal eyes are responsible, are disturbed when the spider cannot see the visual consequences of its own motion.

This can be demonstrated with the simple apparatus shown in Figure 3, which makes use of the spider's ability to hold, walk on, and turn a small card ring of its own weight. The animal is suspended by a small piece of rigid card waxed to the prosoma; this suspension keeps the body stationary in space, although the legs can still move normally relative to the body. Stimuli, usually black dots on a white background, are then presented to the animal, and the kinds of turn that result under these visually open-loop conditions can be studied either by cinematography or by using a matching-pointed system to monitor the angular position of the ring (Land, 1971). It is an interesting comment on the inflexibility of spider behavior that the animals fail to react in any obvious way to the incongruity that results from interchanging a movable ring for the fixed world but will continue for many hours to make logically correct though totally inappropriate movements.

When a small spot is moved a short distance (1 to 5°) in the field of view of the lateral eyes, but outside that of the principal eyes, the spider executes a single rapid turn

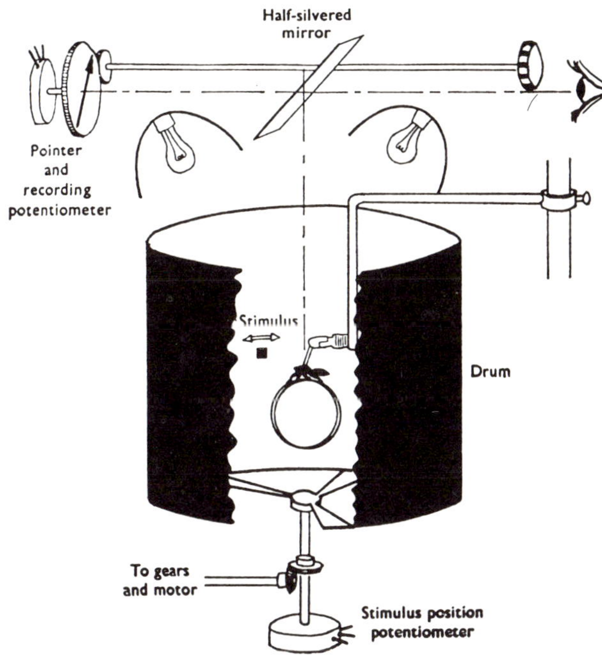

FIGURE 3 Apparatus used to evoke turns in a visually open-loop situation. The spider is fixed in the center of a 12 cm drum and turns its ring when the stimulus is moved a short distance. Stimulus position and angle turned are measured with 360° potentiometers.

whose magnitude is nearly equal to the angle between the stimulus and the body axis: i.e., the angle turned is that which would be required by a free spider to bring the stimulus into the field of vision of the principal eyes (Figure 4). However, the fact that this turn does not result in a change in the relative position of the stimulus demonstrates that, like a human saccade, the size of the turn is dictated in advance solely by the retinal location of the stimulus image. Interesting questions are thus raised about the mechanism of translation between the input of the system (retinal location) and output (stepping leg movements). During a turn the spider steps forward with the legs on one side and backward with those on the other, thereby spinning round within its own length. The accuracy of turning is independent of both the speed of turning (over a tenfold range) and the inertial load (over at least a three-hundredfold range), and so also are the lengths of the steps the spider makes. It seems likely, therefore, that the size of the turn to be made is specified by the retina in terms of the number of steps to be taken: In *Metaphidippus harfordi* each step rotates the animal by approximately 9°, which is a small enough quantum to account for the observed accuracy of turning (Land, 1972).

When a stimulus lies within the field of view of the principal eyes, the situation is quite different. Stationary stimuli are now capable of evoking turns, and under open-loop conditions the visual response to a spot or line 10 to 30° from the body axis is a series of up to 10 small turns, each of about 10°, separated by approximately 100 msec intervals (Figure 5). These turns are very similar to the *Tantalus-like* saccadic pursuit movements made by the human eye when a stabilized image is presented a few degrees away from the fovea (Robinson, 1965). By comparison with turns initiated by the lateral eyes, the control system now operating is formally a closed one (because opening the visual loop results in multiple turns). However, the essential difference between the two systems is simply that the principal eyes, being movable, can detect stationary objects whereas the lateral eyes cannot: A *continuously* moving stimulus presented to the lateral eyes evokes Tantalus-like turning also. Both systems can be said to be of the *sampled data* rather than *continuously monitored* type, but the restrictions on the way data are sampled are different in the two cases.

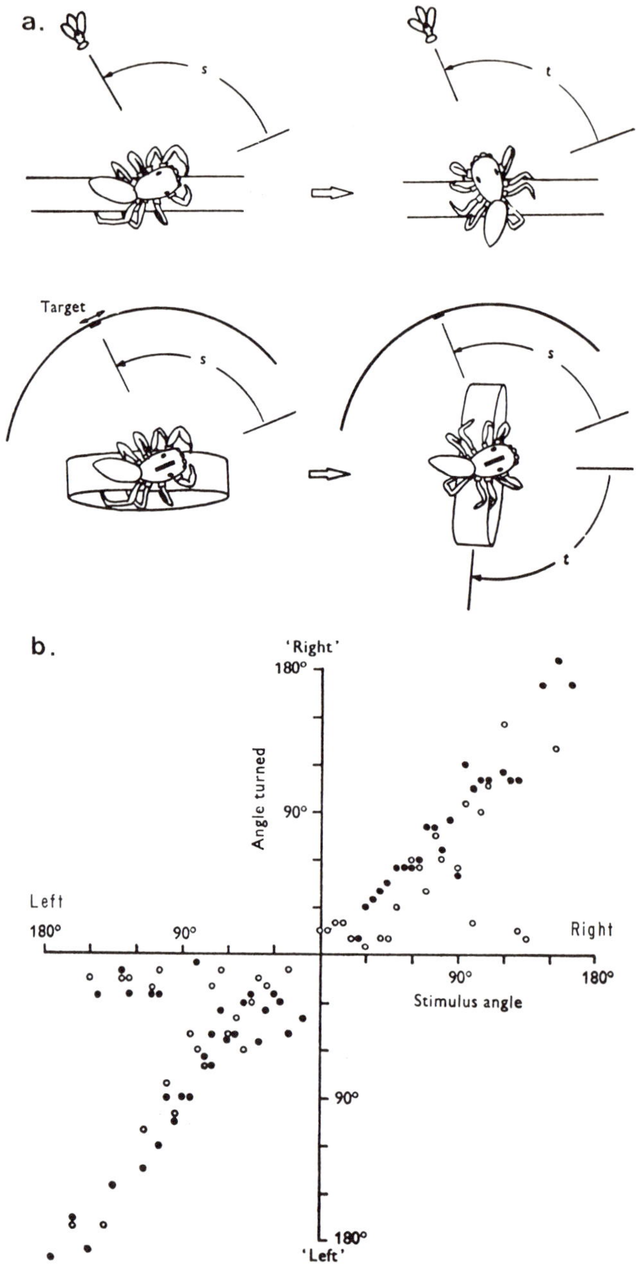

FIGURE 4 (a) *Upper row*: Spider standing on a twig, turning toward a fly 110° to its left. *Lower row*: Open-loop situation in which the spider sees a stimulus 110° to its left and turns the ring through the same angle in the opposite direction. The spider makes the same leg movements as in the upper figure. (b) Result of a single experiment using the apparatus shown in Figure 3. The stimulus was a 5° black spot moved through 5° at 72 different positions around the animal. Most of the points show that the spider makes a turn in which amplitude is nearly equal to the angle the stimulus makes with the animal's body axis. A small proportion of the turns are in the correct direction but are of small amplitude (10 to 20°), which is independent of stimulus position. Free spiders also make both kinds of turn. Open and filled circles indicate stimuli moving in opposite directions.

Eye movements

Perhaps the most extraordinary parallel between jumping spiders and mammals is the finding that the retinae of the principal eyes can be moved with the same three degrees of freedom as the human eye (Land, 1969b). When examined ophthalmoscopically (Figure 6), the retinae are

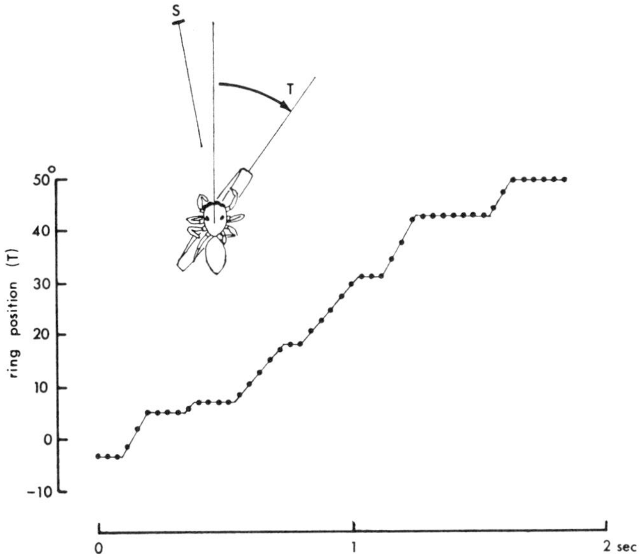

FIGURE 5 "Tantalus-like" turning toward a 2° wide stripe that is stationary, 10° to the left of the spider's axis. The points show the position of the ring on successive frames of film, with the spider in the apparatus shown in Figure 3. This is a fairly typical outcome in which the spider makes 6 turns, whose mean size is 9°, separated by variable intervals of around 100 msec. Multiple turning to stationary stimuli is only seen when the stimulus lies within the field of the movable principal eyes.

seen to move vertically and horizontally, or with a vector combination, and also to rotate about the visual axes by up to 25° in each direction. However, in contrast to the human eye, only the retina and eye tube move, the lens remains fixed so that the retina scans a stationary image. The muscles that move the eyes were first described by Scheuring in 1913; his description was confirmed by Land (1969b). Interestingly, the oculomotor nerve to each eye contains only 6 axons—1 per muscle—which contrasts with man where there are about 10^3 oculomotor axons.

The four kinds of eye movements that have been observed are shown diagrammatically in Figure 7. When the spider is looking at a 30° homogeneous Maxwellian field of view, the eyes make intermittent movements, usually to-and-fro in the horizontal plane but at very varying velocities. These movements can easily be observed in young transparent spiders without ophthalmoscopy, as Dzimirski showed in 1959. These are termed *spontaneous activity* for want of any precise information about their function. If a small dot (1°) is brought into the field of view of either the principal eyes or the anterolateral eyes, the principal retinae move rapidly toward the dot and fixate it with their central regions. The retinal fields of view do not overlap (as in mammals) but are nearly contiguous, as in Figure 7. This movement can be termed a saccade, because it is exactly equivalent to its analogue in humans. If, following fixation, the dot is moved, the retinae will track it with a movement that looks like smooth pursuit, although it would be premature to say more about the control system of tracking at this stage. However, it is clear that when tracking, say a fly, a combination of eye movements (when the stimulus is within 10° of the axis) and small turns by the animal as discussed above are used cooperatively in maintaining fixation when the stimulus strays further from the axis.

The most interesting kind of eye movement is scanning, which occurs after a stimulus has been fixated and is no longer moving (Figure 8). It consists of a very regular oscillatory side-to-side motion of both retinae, from one edge of the stimulus to the other, with a period of 1 to 2 sec. Simultaneously, both retinae rotate about their visual axes by up to 25° in each direction. This movement is also repeated, but the period is much longer (5 to 15 sec). Scanning appears to be a very fixed and experimentally repeatable activity: It has been observed now in 5 species, and no discernable difference was found in its form from one to another. The duration of scanning varies greatly, from bouts lasting longer than a minute to ones consisting of only one or two side-to-side movements; a spider that has been presented with the same spot many times may simply make a saccade toward it and then allow the eyes to drift slowly back to the resting position without scanning at all. The only aspect of scanning that has been found to be affected consistently by the nature of the stimulus is the amplitude of the side-to-side movements: These increase from a minimum of about 1° to a maximum of 10° as the width of the stimulus increases. With stimuli larger than 10°, the retinae tend to drift across the image scanning each edge sequentially.

Although both saccades and tracking movements have obvious counterparts in mammalian vision, scanning appears to be unique. It is true that humans, for example, move their eyes a great deal while examining the visual world and learn to scan in quite specialized ways such as during reading. However, we have here a single very fixed kind of behavior, which appears to be a general purpose procedure for extracting certain important features from the stimulus being scrutinized. What these features may be is discussed in the next section.

Pattern recognition

Jumping spiders are repeatedly faced with the problem of deciding whether the small moving object to which they have just oriented is potential prey or another jumping spider: The importance of getting this decision right is obvious. The moment at which this decision is made is easily determined by an observer; because when con-

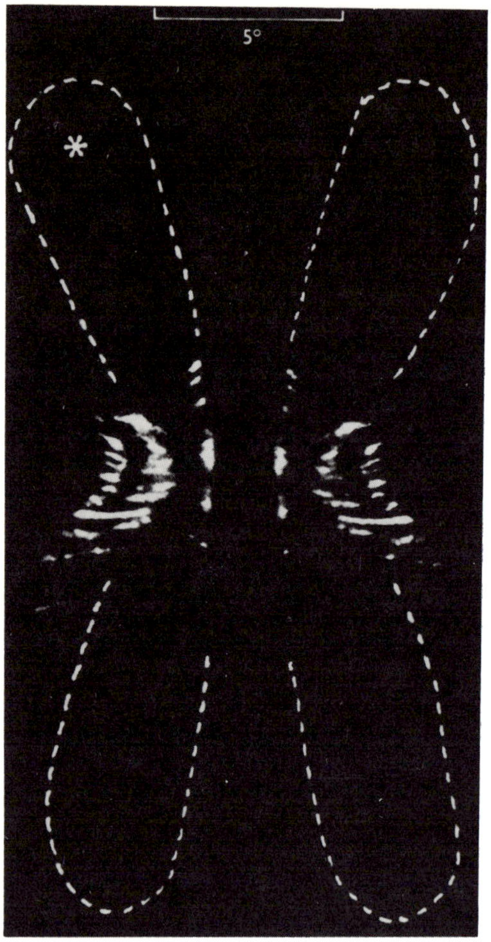

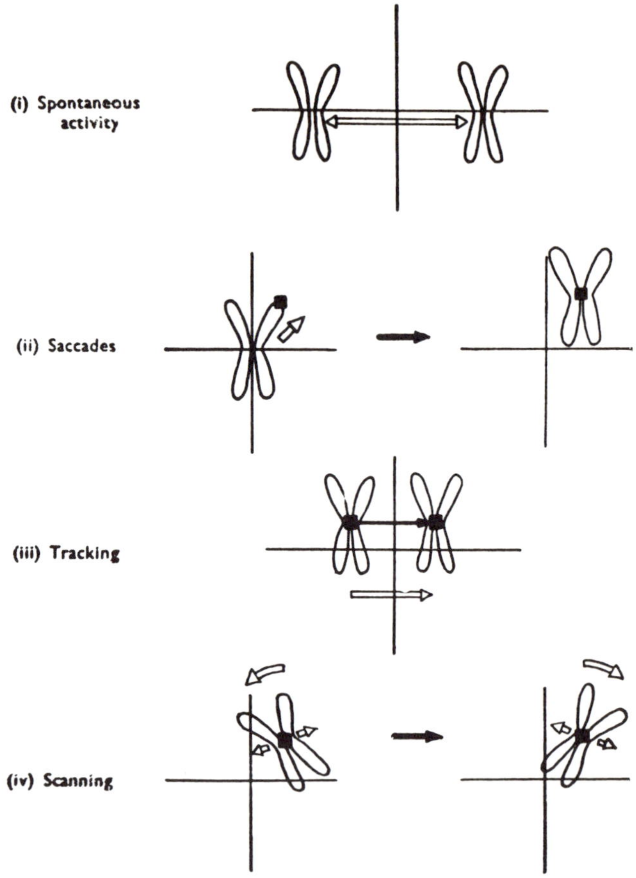

FIGURE 6 Ophthalmoscopic appearance of the retinae of the principal eyes at rest. The photograph was taken with the instrument described in Land (1969b); only the uppermost layer of each retina is visible, and the dotted outline of the rest of the retinae has been reconstructed from the histological structure. The ophthalmoscopic image has the geometrical configuration of the retinal fields of view, which are reversed and inverted with respect to the anatomical layout of the retinae in the body. Note that the fields of view are nearly contiguous but do not overlap. The asterisk (*) corresponds to the ventral region of the right retina.

FIGURE 7 Movements made by the retinae of the principal eyes, (i) without, and (ii - iv) with a stimulus object in the field of view. See text for further details.

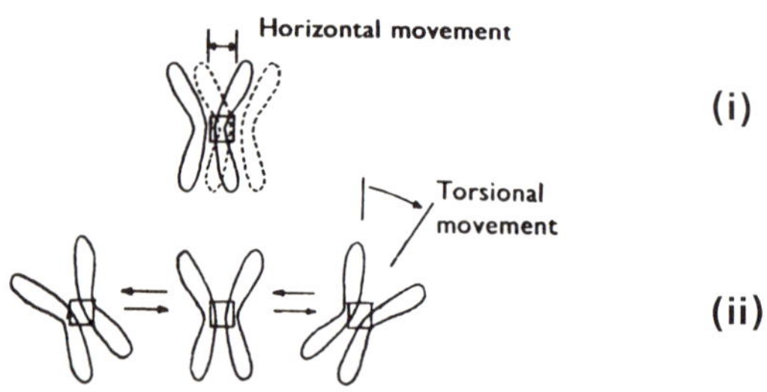

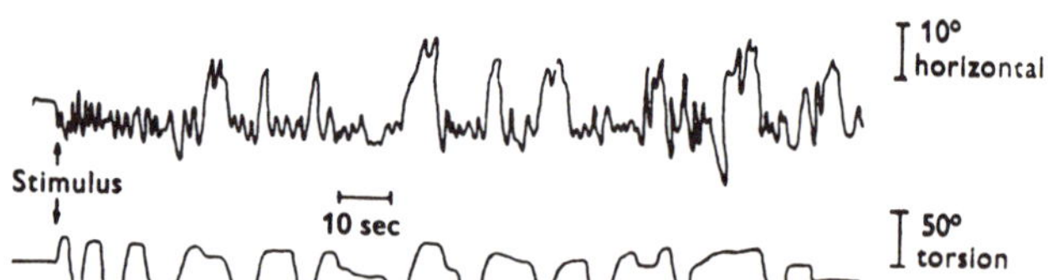

FIGURE 8 Recording of a long bout of "scanning" made using a recording technique in which a movable graticule line is used to track the position and orientation of the inner edge of one of the retinae (Figure 6), while the retina is scanning a 3° dot 5° to the left of the body axis. Scanning consists of a regular side-to-side motion of both retinae (upper trace), coupled to a much slower conjugate rotation (lower trace). After the first 20 sec, scanning becomes irregular and intermittent, merging into spontaneous activity after about a minute. This is an unusually long bout.

fronted with a conspecific, the male spider's behavior changes from a slow approach toward the other animal into a sexual display. In adults this can be quite elaborate, usually involving raising the first pair of legs and proceeding in a series of sideways zigzag arcs that maximize visibility, rather than minimize it as in the slow approach toward prey (for descriptions of salticid sexual behavior see Crane, 1949, or Bristowe, 1958).

Since jumping spiders will display at each other when in separate airtight transparent containers, vision is the only sense involved at least until contact is made, and several workers (Heil, 1936; Crane, 1949; Drees, 1952) have attempted to define what aspects of the visual pattern that one spider presents to another are crucial for recognition. The most thorough analysis is that of Drees; one of his most convincing series of results is shown in Figure 9.

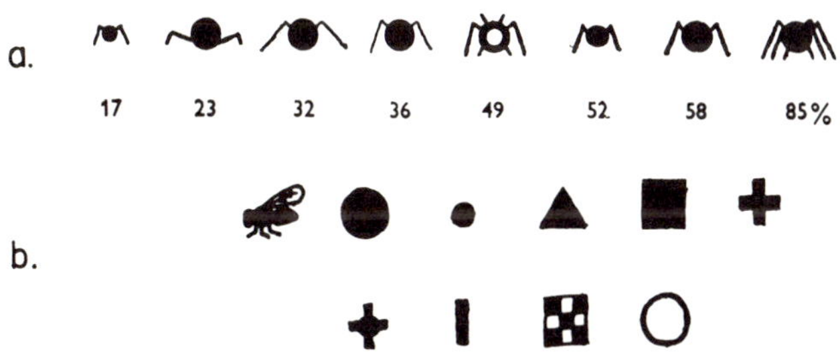

FIGURE 9 One of a series of experiments performed by Drees on *Epiblemum* (*Salticus*) to test which features of a two-dimensional stimulus a male jumping spider would respond to by sexual display, as opposed to preycatching behavior. (a) Figures responded to with sexual display, in order of effectiveness: An ideal "spider" has a number of lines, inclined to the vertical, on each side of a central body. The numbers are the percentages of presentations on which males responded to the figures with a sexual display. (b) All these figures evoked prey capture when moved. (Both figures are after Drees, 1952.)

He found that many different kinds of small object, provided that they had been moved and seen by the spider, elicited prey capture, but that sexual behavior required a rather specific configuration of the object with a central "body" and a pattern of lines—"legs"—on either side. Not surprisingly the optimal pattern obtained by Drees is that most reminiscent of a spider, but it is notable that this two-dimensional, very simplified pattern was almost as effective as a real spider.

From this evidence it is reasonably certain that what the spider is "looking for" during scanning is the presence of lines or edges with appropriate orientations in the target that has been fixated. Let us assume that receptors in the principal retinae are connected centrally in rows, forming line detectors with properties similar to the "simple" cells of the cat's visual cortex (Hubel and Wiesel, 1959). We can then ask how such detectors should be moved in order to find out whether or not a stationary target contained appropriately oriented lines. The answer would be that the detectors must be moved to and fro to detect the presence of lines and rotated to determine their orientation. These movements correspond exactly with the horizontal and torsional components of scanning (Figure 7). It is interesting that scanning by the spider's principal retinae is the precise converse of the operation that a mammalian physiologist performs in trying to determine the orientation selectivity of a cell in the visual cortex: He moves a line stimulus to-and-fro, rotating it until the optimal orientation for that cell is found.

It is implied in the conclusions reached by Drees and by myself that pattern recognition is strictly limited to the single circumscribed tasks of distinguishing prey (which is small and moving but whose geometry is irrelevant) from conspecifics whose geometry is important. At least two other kinds of object are also discriminated: Predators, which are presumably large and whose image on the retinae increases rapidly in size and to which the spider responds by running away or jumping off its substrate, and stationary objects such as twigs, to which the animal may reach out and climb up, or jump onto. There is also some evidence from Drees and others that jumping spiders can discriminate and avoid certain sorts of prey that have proved distasteful. Nongeometrical cues, such as color, also play a part in the final stages of courtship, at least in some species (Crane, 1949). However, none of this modifies the basic conclusion that pattern recognition in these animals differs markedly from that of mammals in that it consists of going through a set procedure (scanning), which leads to a yes-no answer, as opposed to recognition via complex "gestalts," which must be learned and generalized, as is the case in man and presumably other mammals.

Conclusions

Because catching a fly by stalking is not different in principle from catching a bird or mouse, jumping spiders have evolved a range of visual mechanisms that are remarkably similar to those of predatory higher vertebrates. Chief among these are the following:

1. The use of a combination of open- and closed-loop visual control for locating and keeping the prey centrally fixated as the hunt proceeds. The use of different eyes, one set fixed and one with movable retinae, for the performance of these two functions can be regarded as an evolutionary trick that saves a great deal of space in a necessarily small animal, without compromising optical resolution.

2. The development of a versatile system of retinal movements that not only permits close tracking of targets

but also assists directly in making the vital distinction between prey and other spiders—a task that by extension from man's capacity for pattern recognition one simply assumes to present no problem for a mammalian carnivore.

The differences in behavior that result from the limitations of the arthropod nervous system only become apparent when the spider is taken out of the natural situation to which it is adapted and made to perform tricks in the laboratory. Unlike a cat or primate, the spider apparently cannot comprehend that there is something odd about turning a card ring rather than its own body nor that it is strange that stimuli seen to the side never appear in front as they should (Figure 3). The impression is of an animal very well equipped to do a few things well but unable to vary its repertoire. This conclusion is also confirmed by the ease with which jumping spiders can be made to catch dots on paper or display to very simplified representations of other spiders, as well as by the inflexible scanning procedure used to identify stimuli. However, the behavioral limitations are accompanied by an extraordinary degree of neural economy; as examples, each eye muscle is a single motor unit, and identification of another spider at 10 cm requires the participation of a maximum of about 30 receptors out of a total of less than 2000 in both principal eyes. Thanks to two decades of work on single units in crustacean and insect nervous systems, we are now accustomed to finding single cells in arthropods performing functions that require tens or hundreds in higher vertebrates. Nevertheless, it is interesting to find a similar degree of compression in an animal whose activities so closely resemble those of a mammal.

REFERENCES

Barlow, H. B., 1952. The size of ommatidia in apposition eyes. *J. Exp. Biol.* 29:667–674.

Bizzi, E., and E. V. Evarts, 1971. Central control of movement: Eye movements. *Neurosciences Res. Prog. Bull.* 9(1):36–40.

Bristowe, W. S., 1958. *The World of Spiders.* London: Collins.

Crane, J., 1949. Comparative biology of salticid spiders at Rancho Grande, Venezuela. Part IV. An analysis of display. *Zoologica* 34:159–214.

Drees, O., 1952. Untersuchungen über die angeborenen Verhaltensweisen bei Springspinnen (*Salticidae*). *Z. Tierpsychol.* 9:169–207.

Dzimirski, I., 1959. Untersuchungen über Bewegungssehen und Optomotorik bei Springspinnen (*Salticidae*). *Z. Tierpsychol.* 16:385–402.

Eakin, R. M., and J. L. Brandenburger, 1971. Fine structure of the eyes of jumping spiders. *J. Ultrastruct. Res.* 37:618–663.

Eberle, H., 1967. Cone length and chromatic aberration in the eye of *Lebistes reticulatus. Z. Vergl. Physiol.* 57:172–173.

Heil, K. H., 1936. Beiträge zur Physiologie und Psychologie der Springspinnen. *Z. Vergl. Physiol.* 23:1–25.

Homann, H., 1928. Beiträge zur Physiologie der Spinnenaugen. *Z. Vergl. Physiol.* 7:201–268.

Hubel, D. H., and T. N. Wiesel, 1959. Receptive fields of single neurons in the cat's striate cortex. *J. Physiol. (London)* 148:574–591.

Land, M. F., 1969a. Structure of the principal eyes of jumping spiders in relation to visual optics. *J. Exp. Biol.* 51:443–470.

Land, M. F., 1969b. Movements of the retinae of jumping spiders in response to visual stimuli. *J. Exp. Biol.* 51:471–493.

Land, M. F., 1971. Orientation by jumping spiders in the absence of visual feedback. *J. Exp. Biol.* 54:119–139.

Land, M. F., 1972. Stepping movements made by jumping spiders during turns mediated by the lateral eyes. *J. Exp. Biol.* 57:15–40.

Robinson, D. A., 1965. The mechanics of human smooth pursuit eye movement. *J. Physiol. (London)* 180:569–591.

Scheuring, L., 1913. Die Augen der Arachnoiden, II. *Zool. Jb. (Anat.)* 37: 369–464.

37 Behavior of Neurons

C. A. G. WIERSMA

ABSTRACT At least for identifiable neurons, it is legitimate to talk about their "specific" behaviors. The viewpoint is here exposed and defended that the study of behavior of more complexly reacting interneurons can help to bridge the large gap between neurophysiological and behavioral reactions. The necessity of study at this specific level is pointed out. From examples mainly concerned with reactions to diverse visual stimuli, it is concluded that both *attention* and *memory* mechanisms of the animal as a whole are here not assignable to a single locus but have a diffuse representation, because these mechanisms are part of the behavior of individual interneurons, which have to combine their outputs for actual behavioral events to occur.

Introduction

A PREREQUISITE for the development of scientific principles that can lead to an understanding of natural phenomena is the establishment of valid hierarchical levels. It will be the purpose of this chapter to propose that what may be defined as neuronal behavior is such a level, which can bridge the gap between neurophysiology and psychobiology to an as yet unknown extent. Support for stressing the importance of neuronal behavior over connectivity of networks, synaptology, microanatomy, and the like is provided by studies on single cells. Such studies have shown that the reactions of a unit can be so complex as to defy description in terms of these factors. So many parameters would have to be known to predict the reactions, under all circumstances, of most identified interneurons that this is, as yet, well beyond our reach. However, my thesis is that by studying the behavior of such neurons, the behavior of the animal as a whole becomes more explicable. This view is directly opposed to the one in which neurophysiology is considered to be of little or no relevance to animal behavior. Though acknowledging that neurons can serve as telegraph wires, the latter view implies that neurons might be bypassed if a type of field communication were realized. Indeed, the latter concept is fundamental to the existence of extrasensory perception. It may be that this type of communication does exist and that mechanisms are present in the nervous system that cannot be explained on the basis of neuronal behavior. If so, they will be more readily delineated as failures of the proposed approach become evident.

C. A. G. WIERSMA Division of Biology, California Institute of Technology, Pasadena, California

Cell specificity

The assumption that neurons are individually recognizable and that any given one is present in all *normal* specimens of a given species, or at least in a pure line, is central to the view that neuronal behavior warrants study. This is contradictory to a good deal of evidence from higher mammals, e.g. to the proven existence of *plasticity* in function of nerve cells when their connections are changed by surgical means (see Yoon, 1972). I will try to show later why these objections, which on the surface appear to negate the whole thesis, may not be as fatal as it would seem.

Let me first state a rather obvious tenet: If the nervous system in a certain species has developed to a level that is *optimal* for its needs, the best way to ensure that the offspring will be as successful as the parent stock is to provide them with the same number and functional value of all constituent nervous elements. Of course, genetic variability will lead to differences between individuals; therefore, the question arises how large are these normally. Especially from invertebrate studies, it appears, as was shown in several of the preceding articles and will be reiterated here, that interneurons, even those with remarkably complex functions, can readily be individually recognized in all specimens.

Starting at the anatomical level, it has often been possible to identify a cell on the basis of the location of its cell body or its axon. However, minor deviations in this respect frequently occur; for instance, cross-sections of the abdominal cord of the crayfish, though showing overall similarity, are usually not strictly symmetrical, in that axons differ somewhat both in size and in location. The most extreme example that I have ever observed concerned the two medial giant fibers, which have their cell bodies in the brain and end blindly in the telson ganglion. In this specimen, both fibers ran from the brain in the same half of the ventral cord, one being smaller than the other. Notwithstanding this abnormal anatomical location, each made the correct connections in all ganglia, as far as could be ascertained electrophysiologically and anatomically; obviously the functional setup was only slightly distorted, if at all (see Selverston, this volume, for a more extensive discussion on this general subject).

How far is connectivity, by itself, sufficient to provide for the individuality of a neuron? That it is one important, but not exclusive, factor is readily obvious to any neurophysiologist, though not so much so to some modelers of neural networks. Neuromimes, though they have their uses, are dangerous in disregarding the fact that in any nervous system different types of neurons are present that, by their inherent properties, react quite specifically to their inputs, even though the latter may be identical. This is an important point, because it illustrates the danger of concluding what the functional significance of a presynaptic axon is from its firing pattern. Obviously the result depends both on the type of postsynaptic effect, excitatory or inhibitory, and on the synaptic efficiency. But connectivity in conjunction with transmitter sensitivity is not the whole story involved in neuronal behavior, as other known properties of neurons enter into the picture. The main one of these is the variation in tendency to fire *spontaneously*, an aspect that may be much more widespread than is generally assumed and appears to be present in various preset amounts. It leads to such features as a cell being driven to fire at a higher rate than its spontaneous one by an inhibitory input and the triggering of a number of discharges by a single presynaptic event. In addition, our ever-increasing knowledge of the complexities existing at the synaptic level itself, e.g. synaptic regulation of electrotonic coupling between cells (Bennett and Spira, 1972), presence of excitatory and inhibitory receptive sites sensitive to the same transmitter substance (Kandel, 1968) further illustrates the difficulties in describing input-output relationships in terms of synaptic events. Of course, this does not mean that it would not be worthwhile to determine for any given interneuron class its connectivities and types of presynaptic and postsynaptic influences, as well as its "amount" of spontaneity, and such additional factors as changes in firing level, whether or not hormonally induced. Since several of these variables may involve time factors of considerable duration, long-term changes in reactivity do not necessarily indicate "plastic" properties, in the sense that the cell acquires properties that it would not have had "normally." *Plasticity* becomes very much a question of definition, because different states merge into one another, without sharp boundaries. That neurons can show real plasticity cannot be denied. For instance, the experiments of Yoon (1971, 1972) on the goldfish optic tectum in which he was able to make retinal neurons form reversible connections with different parts of the tectum, by blocking and unblocking its posterior half, clearly demonstrate that interneurons can change their functional connection. This type of finding shows that predetermination as present in all cases of identifiable neurons is not absolute but can be changed by experimental and thus presumably developmental circumstances. It, however, is also indicated that the nervous system is still working on the principle of very deterministic types of interconnectivity, for when only about half of the normal complement of neurons are available, all appear to change, many giving up their normal inputs to make room for those that are "homeless," but in an orderly manner. Since functional recovery of optic reflexes from the retinal part that was disconnected is found, it seems indicated that these arrangements also involve the output channels of the optic tectum cells. These findings can therefore not be considered as in favor of a type of information transmission by whole populations as against cell specific activity.

The study of individual neuronal behavior has as one of its main goals the understanding of how the information flow between inputs and outputs is structured. On the input side one can ask how the firing rate is related to environmental changes. As we will see, this relationship may vary strongly due to factors other than the main input channel. On the output side one can obtain useful information about the significance of a given interneuron by stimulating it directly and observing the effect in terms of overall movements of body parts or of combinations of muscular contractions. Variations in this output due, for instance, to localized sensory stimulation of the body parts involved can further reveal the amount of modulation such programmed motor patterns undergo by local events. In preceding papers of this part, several examples and discussions of this topic have been provided. For interneurons on the sensory side, intracellular stimulation, which has so far been only occasionally used, appears to be much less revealing, because no readily observable output in the form of motor effects results. In such cases, it would therefore be necessary to discover the various interneurons toward the motor side for which such a fiber is presynaptic in order to evaluate its functional significance. Therefore, the study of the reactivity of such fibers to the presynaptic events has been so far the main approach.

Sensory representation in the CNS

An aspect present in invertebrates, which has so far no known equivalent in vertebrates, is the representation of large, mutually overlapping sensory fields, with an apparent absence of restricted fields immediately beyond the primary sensory level. It does appear as if the often quite good resolution present in the periphery due to the many sense cells is not centrally used, but whether this is actually the case is still problematic, because at least one case is known in which very accurate representation of primary sensory input is strongly indicated (see below, page 423). To illustrate the representation of large sensory fields by interneurons, that for the dorsal hairs on the crayfish abdomen may be briefly mentioned (Wiersma and Hughes, 1961; Wiersma and Bush, 1963). The minimum extent of the sensory areas to which the interneurons involved react consists of one-half of each dorsal abdominal segment. In addition there are interneurons responding to two, three, or more successive unilateral areas, some with also a contralateral representation, as well as interneurons with larger bilateral fields culminating in one that is responsive to touch of hairs anywhere on the whole body. As a result, touch of one dorsal abdominal area can activate as many as 20 interneurons. These findings illustrate a pronounced parallel computation of the information for which the functional significance is not immediately obvious. It should be noted that this system is a very poor one for retrieval of more exact stimulus localization, because in this case it could hardly be more precise than that provided by the interneurons with the smallest sensory fields. The likely explanation is that the information carried by the different neurons, which react to one local stimulation, feed into various output channels, causing more localized or widespread reactions, related to their sensory field size. Some evidence for this type of connectivity is indicated for the crayfish abdominal ganglia by the experimental results of Kennedy (1971), and also for visual interneurons as we will see later.

Feature detection by single units

To various degrees, reaction only to specific aspects of a given stimulus situation is provided by specialization of the primary sense cells. Many examples come readily to mind, and I will quote here one case, to illustrate the difficulties involved in deducing the consequences of this type of parallel input. Elastic strand organs in the joints of crustacean appendages have their origin usually on a tendon, and their insertion is either on a hard part of the more distal segment or on the joint membrane. The most peripheral joint of each thoracic appendage is spanned by such a strand, in which the sensory endings of numerous neurons are embedded (Whitear, 1962; Mill and Lowe, 1971). The sensory fibers are divided into four distinct classes; two indicate position in one or the other direction from the midpoint, and two are specifically triggered by movements, one type for each direction. Frequency changes occur in the movement fibers only within a small velocity range, because a "saturation" rate is reached when the velocity is only slightly above threshold; however, the saturation rates may vary with the load (Wiersma et al., 1970). Fibers with different thresholds are present in all classes (Wiersma and Boettiger, 1959; Wiersma, 1959). The total result is that the CNS receives very accurate information about the peripheral situation almost constantly, because both frequency and fiber number coding are available for position, and number coding is available for movement. Though the overall output has been shown to be of importance for the firing patterns of both motor and inhibitory fibers to the muscles moving the joint (Bush, 1965; Spirito et al., 1972), it is as yet not known in which way the different fiber types and the individual ones of each type are involved in the resulting myotatic reflexes. Rather unexpectedly it was found that this input is not of importance to the normal motions of either its own or other legs, as in walking (Barnes et al., 1972). For central fibers responsive to induced joint motions, of which many react to various joints of more than one leg (Wiersma, 1958), it is also unknown whether the position and movement signals are separately channeled or whether these two informational aspects are recombined. Whether different pathways are present for low- and high-threshold events in either type of input is another unsolved problem.

Especially in optic systems, it is certain that feature detection is mainly performed by the neuronal connections in the optic ganglia, though it is difficult to decide to what extent peripheral selectivity and interconnectivity of the primary sense cells are also involved. Photopic, scotopic, and color vision depend on such peripheral differentiation. Lateral inhibition between primary photoreceptors often appears to be present, but at least in some decapods there is, in addition, a similar type of inhibition that depends on neuronal connections. Here, light in an area far outside the excitatory field of an interneuron inhibits, as does light shining in the other eye, and both must depend on a neuronal network. Specific reactivity to movement involves spatial and temporal readout of neuronal collecting stations by neural networks, and it is remarkable that several types of interneurons responsive to movement are present, each optimally reacting to a different aspect of the movement and the physical features of the targets. For instance, in crustacean optic nerves one finds on the one hand the "jittery movement fibers" that react to a black object entering into the field from any direction, but which soon stop firing whenever large objects travel linearly through it. On the other hand, the unidirectional movement fibers usually fire more strongly the farther an object travels linearly in the preferred direction but are inhibited by opposite movements. This example shows that each fiber type has its specific inhibitory mechanism that must be provided by different networks regulating the same input channels. I quote this special instance to illustrate how difficult it may be to determine the connectivity involved in each type.

Table I lists the known types of interneurons reactive to visual stimuli in different species of decapods. Note that certain types of "feature extractors" appear to be present in all species, whereas others have been encountered in only one. Of course, the absence of a class in a species does not necessarily mean that it does not exist, for the methods used do preferentially show fibers of larger diameter. Nevertheless there does appear to be a relationship between the visual behavior of an animal and its visual interneuron equipment. A comparison of the crayfish and rock lobster, whose optic nerves have been studied most, shows that behaviorally the crayfish is visually less "astute," in accord with its fewer optic fiber classes. In a considerable number of insects, the indications are that the neurons in the optic system are very similar to those in the crustaceans, but perhaps because their numbers are much larger, identification of specific interneurons has not been made in most cases. Much current research concerns this problem in insects.

TABLE I

Table of known visual fibers in the different decapod types investigated

Class of Fiber	Crayfishes	Rock Lobsters	Crabs
Sustaining	+	+	+
Dimming	+	+	+
Jittery movement	+	+	+
Light movement		+	
Medium movement		+	+
Fast movement	+ ?	+	+
Seeing		+	?
Slow movement			+
Space constant	+	+	+
Unidirectional movement	+ ?	+	+
Multimodal	+	+	+

(From Wiersma and Yanagisawa, 1971.)

Centrifugal influences

Of the various classes of visually reactive interneurons in the crustacean optic nerve, the sustaining and dimming ones appear to be the "earliest" both with regard to their rather simple type of integration and to their apparently more peripherally located origin in the optic ganglion chain. Nevertheless, their discharges are strongly influenced by centrifugal factors, such as the inhibitory influence from contralateral eye neurons (T. Yamaguchi, personal communication) and the facilitatory effect of the general state of excitement of the animal (Wiersma and Yamaguchi, 1966). An excited state may cause as much as a fivefold increase in the number of impulses elicited by a light flash (Figure 1), although the state by itself does not give rise to impulses during a dark period if no dark discharge is present and can at best raise it to a still low discharge rate (Aréchiga and Wiersma, 1969a). The effect can be pictured as due to a lowering of the threshold at the spiking locus by the excited state, but other explanations such as removal of inhibition are not excluded.

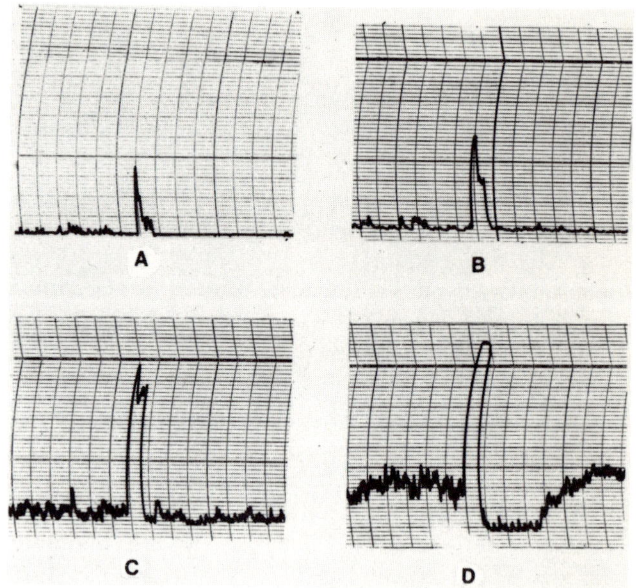

FIGURE 1 Changes in responsiveness of a crayfish sustaining fiber to a constant light stimulus with various states of activity of the animal. The electrode was implanted and the animal had been adapted for several hours to a dim light (0.01 candle/ft^2). A light pulse of 4 candle/ft^2 and of 15 sec duration was applied successively during an experiment of several minutes duration. In (A) the animal was in a "sleep" attitude. In (B) it walked slowly in its container. In (C) the animal was more aroused by external mechanical stimuli, and in (D) it was in a "defense reflex" position, ready for attack. Note that the frequency of the background discharge to the low light level also increases with the state of excitement. (From Aréchiga and Wiersma, 1969a.)

It is interesting to note that light shining on the eye can bring about a higher state of excitement, but this may take up to a few seconds, whereas an increase of excited state causes an almost immediate increase in the visual response. A possible centrifugal pathway causing this increase is provided by the so-called activity fibers, whose discharge rate is proportional to the excited state level (Figure 2). Again, this mechanism is inferred and needs experimental confirmation of the predicted increase of sustaining fiber discharge on electrical stimulation of the activity fiber. Since it is possible to implant electrodes

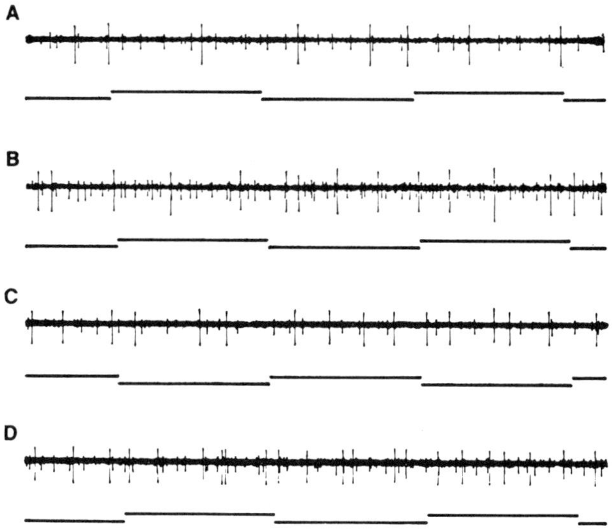

FIGURE 2 Illustration of the relationship in firing frequency between a centrifugal interneuron (small spikes) and a sustaining fiber (large spikes) during different levels of excitement and light intensity in a crayfish. (A) Low light level stimulus during a low state of excitement. The smaller centrifugal "activity fiber" fires at the same rate as it would in total darkness (12 impulses per sec). The sustaining fiber for the back upper rim (038) gives a sustained discharge of 4 impulses per sec. In (B) the light level was identical, but the state of excitement was increased by mechanical stimulation. The firing rate of the activity fiber increased to 28 impulses per sec, that of 038 to 8 per sec; both fibers fired therefore about two times more frequently. Here (C) and (D) are records of the same preparation at a later time, and with an increased light level. In (C) the 038 fires at a sustained rate of 7 per sec although the activity level is about the same as in (A), as indicated by the activity fiber that again fires at 12 per sec. In (D) this rate is 22 per sec (lower than in B) and 038 fires at 11 per sec. The percent increase in either is therefore less than from (A) to (B), however, the ratio is somewhat less similar. In (A) and (C) the tethered preparation showed no movements of the appendages, in (B) and (D) they were pronounced. (From Wiersma and Yamaguchi, 1967.)

that remain functional for extended periods of time (e.g. 1 month) (Aréchiga and Wiersma, 1969b), such experiments appear feasible.

While it is known that the excited state influences both sustaining and dimming fibers in the same way, its influence on the firing rates of other optic fiber classes appears to be much less, and not present in all. In the rock lobster, several of the fiber classes are, instead, specifically regulated by other factors. This is especially well illustrated by the seeing fibers (Wiersma and York, 1972). These interneurons are more complex in that their excitatory field boundaries, though in most instances not much different from those in the simpler classes, are vague and not necessarily the same for objects traveling in opposite directions. An additional feature is that the field consists of two distinguishable but not distinct parts, one in which a moving target is perceived but no reaction to a stationary one occurs, and a more central area in which a stationary object also causes impulses for as long as 30 sec. These fibers seem to be clearly influenced by the "mood" of the animal in that they have a low reactivity when the animal is "drowsy," react well when the animal is in a waking state, and are actually inhibited if the animal is in a high state of excitement, as during a defense reaction. On the other hand, in this situation, but not during walking, the jittery movement fibers are highly sensitive and their normally high rate of habituation decreases greatly. It is not difficult to conjecture reasons for these differences when the behavior of the animal is considered. Seeing fibers are almost certainly the input pathways for the pointing reactions of the lobster's antennae that consist of rather accurately tracking a target, e.g. a fish (Lindberg, 1955), because the habituation of the pointing reflex and that of the seeing fibers to the same object often coincide; furthermore, both habituations can often be negated by moving the target through another trajectory. On the other hand, one specific jittery movement fiber most likely triggers and others sustain the defense reflex, as will be discussed next. Therefore the difference in behavior of the seeing and the jittery movement fibers under different circumstances relates well with their final output tasks.

The specific jittery movement fiber mentioned belongs to a special set of visual interneurons, the space-constant ones, of which one member occurs in the majority of the classes. The space-constant fibers have in common that in the normal eye position they respond to stimuli above the eye's horizontal axis and to a symmetrical field on the lower eye half when the animal is in the upside-down position. In many, but not all cases, the potential field encompasses the whole retina. Their maximum field size occurs when the middle of the potential field points straight upward (Figure 3). This control by gravity is mainly provided by the statocysts, and because their removal results in the sensory field becoming of maximal size even when the eye points downward, the influence is obviously inhibitory. We have here a good example of one input channel that is read out by a number of otherwise quite differently behaving interneurons. It, of course, also indicates that this space-constant mechanism is of great importance to the animal, presumably for spatial localization. Since the sizes of the visual fields change very accurately with statocyst position, the channel transmitting the information has to consist of the axons of the primary sense cells of that organ, and indications that these do, indeed, reach the optic ganglia have been obtained. Thus here is a case in which the accuracy of the primary sensory input appears to be used to its fullest extent.

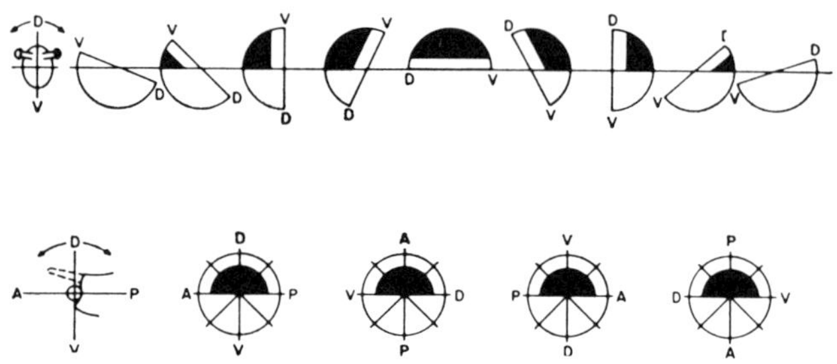

FIGURE 3 Illustration of how the field of a crayfish space-constant sustaining fiber travels over the surface of the eye as body position is changed. In (A) the animal was rotated along its longitudinal axis, and the sustaining fiber ceased to respond as soon as every part of its visual field looked at objects below the horizon, whereas the field was enlarged and circular when its whole potential field was exposed to light from above. In (B) the animal was rotated about its transverse axis, in which case the visual field did not change in extent, but rotated in the opposite direction over the eye surface. (From Wiersma and Yamaguchi, 1967.)

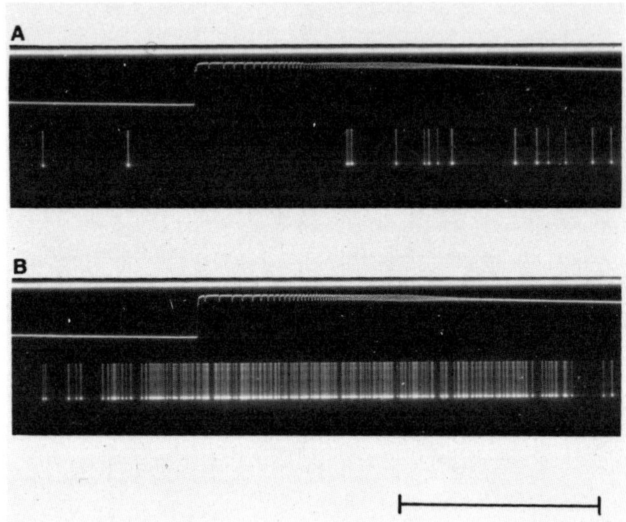

FIGURE 4 Rock lobster seeing fiber looking at moving targets of different dimensions and reacting distinctly different to them. The seeing fiber used was LO 141, which has a rather complex binocular visual field. In (A) the visual stimulus was a vertical stripe made up of 5 black squares (15°) traveling at a speed of 8° per sec through the field. This led to an inhibition of its background discharge rate. In (B) only the middle of the 5 squares was left in place. With the same rotation speed, there was now a strong discharge as soon as the target entered the field, which remained until it left. Time base, 5 sec. The upper lines monitor both drum speed and position; the sudden jump occurs at one constant drum position. (Spike events were transcribed from tape to Grass polygraph by a spike height selective transducer.) (From Wiersma and York, 1972.)

Attention

The seeing fibers show a number of features that can be described in psychological terms. This does not mean, for instance, that when a seeing fiber pays attention to a particular object that the *animal* itself does so. Under several circumstances the seeing fibers can completely neglect an object when introduced in their visual field. When an object enters and travels very slowly through the field it will not elicit any impulses from either the movement or the seeing area. When interesting visual stimuli occur in other eye regions during a "seeing" reaction, they often lead to a severe reduction in spike number, and the frequency may then increase again when the distracting stimulus stops. Another aspect of this type of inhibition is that while a moving target larger than the visual field may be ignored, reduction of its size can, on the next turn, give a vigorous discharge (Figure 4). At least some of the seeing fibers can be similarly "distracted" by purely mechanical stimulation, for instance, in the case of a seeing fiber looking in the forward direction, by stroking the animal's tail. However, an enhancement of this fiber's discharge can be obtained by appropriate movements of the antenna. One category of unidirectionally sensitive fibers was very reactive when an object moved over the "entrance" part of the field at a rather slow rate. Passage over the rest of the field would then give a strong response, but when the entrance part was quickly traversed, the response for the remainder of the field stayed low even for the speed that was optimal under the first condition. One may describe this as the presence of a trigger zone for attention.

Memory

The seeing fibers possess a short-term memory mechanism, which has been shown in two ways: One is to turn out the light while the fiber is giving a "seeing" discharge. It will then resume firing when the target is reilluminated, e.g. after 10 sec, but will be silent if the target has been removed in the dark. Conversely, when a target is placed in the seeing area during a dark period, the fiber will start to fire shortly after illumination, but only when the dark period is not longer than about 30 sec (Figure 5) (Wiersma and York, 1972).

A longer lasting and less distractable memory-like phenomenon is exhibited by the motor neurons that effect horizontal optokinetic movements of the outer eyecup. The discovery of such a memory mechanism was made in the crab, *Carcinus*, by Horridge (1965, 1966, 1968) who registered eyecup position. This was studied in considerable detail by Shepheard (1966), under stimulus conditions much like those we are now using. Our results agree fairly well for such factors as duration of memory. We have shown that the motor fibers of the rock lobster, which are driven by optokinetic input, are responsible for the phenomenon (York et al., 1972). The input for the optokinetic reaction is normally elicited by turns performed by the animal (though this is contrary to the view that only passive and not active turns elicit them) (Dijkgraaf, 1956) and is mimicked by turning a striped drum around the animal. In the crayfish the read-in for this reflex appears to be provided by two unidirectional movement fibers, responding antagonistically, that discharge only during motion. In the rock lobster on the other hand, two fibers with similar fields, also apparently located in the optic nerve, differ from those of the crayfish in that they, like the optokinetic motor fibers, show afterdischarges when movement stops. And besides the difference in localization, they are strictly responsive to ipsilateral input (York et al., 1972), whereas the motor fibers are usually reactive to both eyes. Unfortunately, it is therefore still uncertain which interneurons are involved in the optokinetic reflex.

All evidence, however, is against making the same input pathways responsible for both the optokinetic reflex and the memory read-in and read-out. We found that the memory, if any, was poor for a moving object; i.e., if stripes have been turning for some time when the light is turned off, their position at light "off" is not remembered. When stripes are turned during a dark period and the light is turned on up to 5 min after it went off, appropriate and clear positive or negative responses are often obtained (Figure 6). This is one reason why movement fibers as such cannot be regarded as the source for the input,

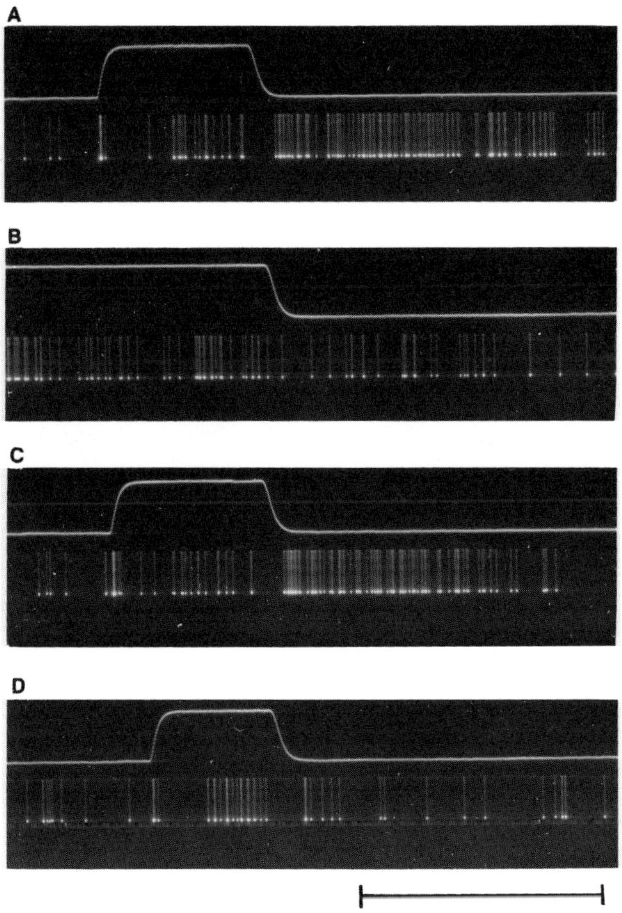

FIGURE 5 Memory response of a binocular seeing fiber (LO 121) of the rock lobster. A target (15° square) was placed or omitted in the seeing area of the fiber during periods of darkness, indicated by the upward deflection of the upper signal, monitoring light intensity. In (A) and (C), the target was introduced during a 3-sec dark period, and the fiber responded strongly to this situation when the light was turned on. In (B) the dark period was started 19 sec before the light was turned on and, notwithstanding the target's presence, no significant discharge resulted after relighting. In other instances the "memory-span" of a seeing fiber was found to be somewhat longer but did not exceed 30 sec in duration. In (D) no target was placed in the drum and no discharge resulted from relighting. (From Wiersma and York, 1972.)

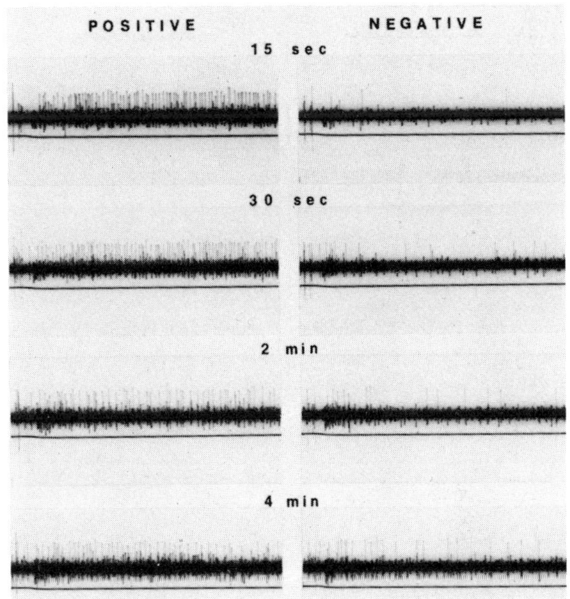

FIGURE 6 "Memory-span" of an horizontal optokinetic motor fiber of the shore crab, *Pachygrapsus crassipes*. The animal was in the center of a striped drum (stripe width was 12°), in which it was left at least 1 min before the light was turned out for 5 sec. During this dark time, the drum was rotated by 3°, either in the positive (that is, the direction that would increase the fiber's discharge when drum was turned in the light) or in the negative direction. The latter would silence the fiber except when a fast nystagmic eye motion occurred, when it would give a short burst. The left column shows a gradual decrease in the positive direction, as the period of darkness increased from 15 sec to 4 min; the right-hand column, a more or less corresponding increase in spike events. Significant differences between positive and negative results can be present for times somewhat exceeding 5 min. Lower lines, light intensity. Each record starts just before light is turned on. (Each record is 12½ sec long.) (Wiersma and Hirsh, unpublished.)

because they do not react to any extent under these conditions. Not only stripes but also randomly distributed targets can elicit both reflex and memory.

In an as yet unpublished series of experiments performed on optokinetic motor fibers with Dr. Hirsh and the late Dr. Reddy, it was found that the maximum angle of a dark turn giving rise to a positive or negative read-out depends on the stripe width. No read-out occurs when the drum is moved one stripe width, and from this point on the effect becomes negative for positive turns and the reverse (Figure 7). The minimum angle of rotation that gave rise to positive responses was somewhat different for the species used. In the lobster it is about 0.4°, in the crayfish 0.2°, and 0.1° in the shore crab (Table II). In all cases this resolution is far better than would be indicated by the angle neighboring ommatidia make with each other.

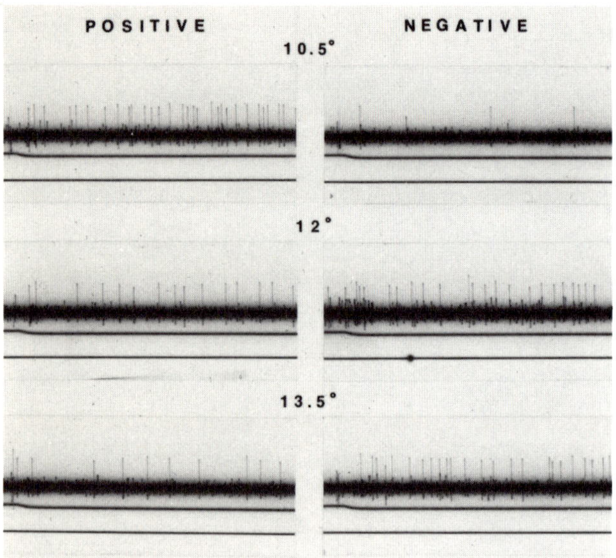

FIGURE 7 Reversal point for positive as against negative memory read-out for an optokinetic motor fiber, for 12° wide stripes, in *Pachygrapsus*. When turned in the dark period (5 sec) for 10.5° the read-out is positive for a positive turn, but at 13.5° it is negative. Negative turns show the reverse. At 12° the two turns give the same result. If the stripes were 6° wide, a turn of that value would give the "undecided" answer. Each record is 12½ sec long. (Wiersma and Hirsh, unpublished.)

The eyes can be prevented from changing position in the crab and crayfish by gluing them to the carapace. With regard to the duration of the memory and the minimum angle, the results were very similar to those obtained from the same fiber before this procedure. However, the duration of the change in discharge was invariably longer when the eyes were fixed. This phenomenon is difficult to explain, because the moving eye would counteract the discharge when it moved in the right direction, but back-

TABLE II
Visual acuity in Pachygrapsus

Angle of Turn	Number of Spikes		Difference
	Positive	Negative	Pos. − Neg.
1.6°	87	2	85
0.8°	59	15	44
0.4°	43	7	36
0.2°	34	4	30
0.1°	32	9	23
0.05°	16	—	—

Protocol: 12° stripes turned in indicated direction during 5 sec dark period; spikes counted during 5 sec period after light on.

drift, as indicated by the gradual decrease in frequency, should enhance the discharge duration, because this would constitute a positive stimulus. Therefore, in the moving eye the frequency should be lower at first, which appears to be so, but should subsequently decrease only gradually, whereas in reality it stops considerably sooner than in the glued eye (Figure 8).

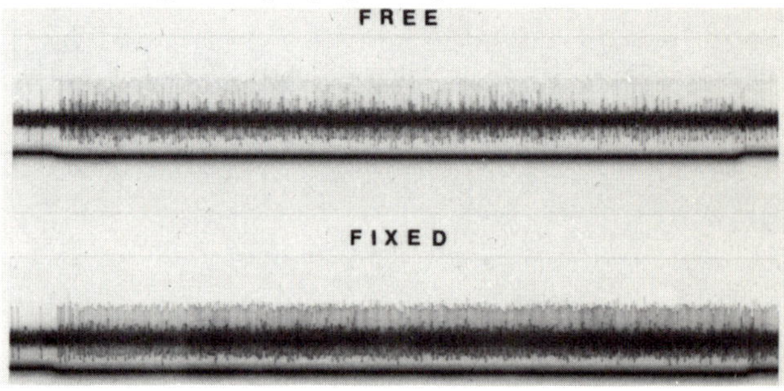

FIGURE 8 Comparison of read-out of the same optokinetic motor fiber in *Pachygrapsus*, before and after the eye was made immobile by gluing it to the carapace. A 3° turn was given during darkness in the positive direction for the fiber. The lower line shows the moment when light went on (and off after 20 sec). Note that read-out starts at the same time, is somewhat weaker in the beginning for the free eye, and remains at considerably higher frequency in the fixed one. Record durations, 25 sec. (Wiersma and Hirsh, unpublished.)

We did not obtain any strong effects of eye drift during the dark period. The three species differ with regard to the effect of darkness on the firing frequency. In the rock lobster the basic frequency is regularly lower in the dark than in light and, therefore changes, especially after dark turns in the positive direction. Both decreases and increases occur in the crab during darkness, whereas in the crayfish increases are usually obtained, so that negative turns are then often especially effective. We found that excited states and even eye withdrawal reflexes elicited during darkness are in general compatible with the correct amount of subsequent read-out, and we have practically never encountered read-outs that after these procedures were of the opposite sign from those expected. This is remarkable, especially for the rock lobster where the large changes in frequency for positive turns are present, notwithstanding that there must have been eye drift during the low-frequency dark discharge. Note that in this respect our results differ from those of Shepheard (1966) who frequently found reversed eye movements after longer dark periods. Dark discharge rates thus appear to be unrelated to the memory process, one reason to exclude afterimages as reference points for the read-out. Another reason for rejecting a peripheral location of the memory mechanism is that the intensity of the read-out is relatively independent of the read-in and read-out illumination levels. Furthermore, the strongest afterimage should be caused by the overhead light, which, because it was often as much as 20° from vertical, would change in position with regard to the eye only when the animal is turned within the drum. Experiments in which drum versus animal turning by equal amounts were compared usually showed no noticeable differences and therefore the afterimage of the light was not used as a reference point.

It should be realized that the memory input needs the stimulation of a number of collecting stations in order to be effective. For instance, a single black stripe will give at best a weak effect, whereas three black stripes are nearly as effective as a completely striped surround, even when widely separated. When such stripes were built from single square targets (15°) and subsequently distributed randomly within the same surface area, it was found that the responses were equivalent. If, afterwards, the number of targets was reduced to that of a single stripe, distributed over the sum total surface area, the reduced result was equivalent to that of a single stripe. This shows that the read-in stations in horizontal movements summate their reactions and that each contributes about equally whether distributed over the total surface area of the eye or arranged in stripes.

Read-in Times By letting the animal look for preset times at a stationary background, it can be decided how long it takes before memory is established. This process is not all or none, and, as shown by Shepheard (1966), varies with the length of exposure. In *Carcinus*, maximal responses to small angles require a relatively long period of up to 70 sec. In our experience 60 sec read-in is only slightly better than 30 sec, but shorter times decrease the response. We have used another approach to determine this factor. After a new situation was exposed for a given number of seconds, it was noted whether a second turn in the opposite direction would give an appropriate discharge to the shortly exposed position or would still signal this final position in relation to the first, well read-in situation. Two main variations have been used. In one, the drum was turned 3° in either direction and then turned back to the original position. Under these circumstances, the read-out would either be appropriate for the second turn or no effect would ensue if read-in had failed. The minimum read-in times thus found were usually quite short, especially in the crab, where appropriate responses appeared with exposures as short as one second. In the second method, the second turn was only half the size of the first, again in the opposite direction (Figure 9). Here the final result can be still of the same sign as the first, because with regard to the original situation the stripe position had changed, though less, in the same

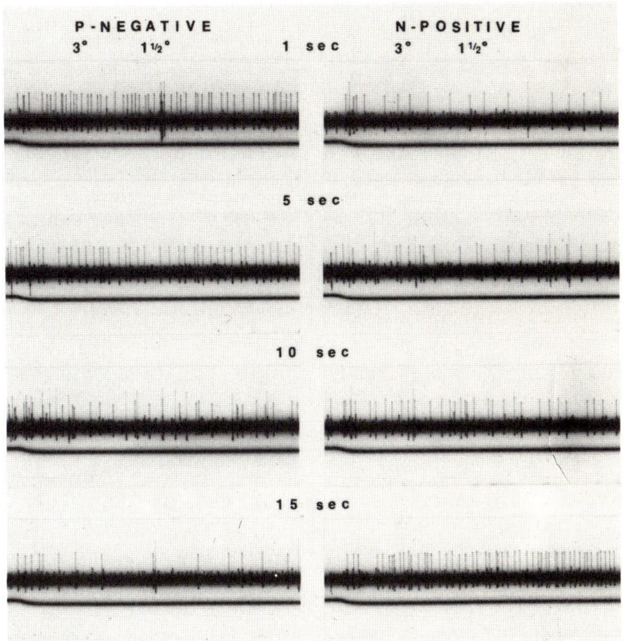

Figure 9 Read-in time of a 12° striped pattern after it was moved from a stationary position to which the eye had been exposed for 60 sec as determined by the read-out after a second turn in the opposite direction, following various exposure times. The second turn was only half that of the first, so that with insufficient read-in time the displacement is referred to the direction of the first turn (original memory) and is in the direction of the second turn, when the "new" memory is sufficiently read in. The record shows that the "old" and the "new" memories are mutually antagonistic. Where the second turn is negative (first column) the read-out after only 1 sec exposure is still positive and is not clearly negative until 15 sec of exposure. The reverse is true when the first turn was negative and the second positive (second column). At 10 sec there was no significant read-out. Of the two read-outs, only the one after the second turn is shown. Lower signal, light on after second dark turn. Each record is 15 sec in length. (Wiersma and Hirsh, unpublished.)

direction, or it can be reversed in sign, when the second position is sufficiently read-in. As expected, a longer time was needed before a reversal occurred, varying from $2\frac{1}{2}$ sec to as long as 15 sec. We often observed that these times increased during an experimental session, indicating a weakening of the memory mechanism. Such loss of memory can become total, when the mechanism deteriorates presumably due to oxygen lack, at a time when the optokinetic reflex discharges are still quite strong. In lobsters we have met with some individuals who seemed to lack optomotor fiber memory, though they were apparently in excellent condition; we have also seen lobsters that lost this memory after a few sessions but regained it after several weeks rest. I mention these facts because, although hardly solid data, they do indicate that memory and optokinetic mechanisms are different and also that afterimages are not likely to be the basic mechanism involved in memory.

Localization of the memory mechanism may be difficult. One fact is evident: Because there is a marked difference between the read-out of a driving eye against that of one being driven by the other's input, each seems to have its own mechanism with a weaker connection to the other eye. However, there may be a total of four memory locations. For, although the output is usually symmetrical, in that positive and negative responses are of similar magnitude for dark turns in opposite directions, in several animals either excitation or inhibition was clearly more pronounced, pointing to two memory locations, one for each direction.

It is clear that these are useful systems for further study, but how far the phenomenon can be resolved to its fundamental processes remains speculative. However, some worthwhile conclusions are evident from Shepheard's (1966) and our results. One is that there is competition between the old and the new memory, so read-in is not an all-or-none phenomenon. Another is that this memory system is present in most animals to an equivalent extent, and that it occurs under circumstances that are more comparable to those involved in imprinting than in most learning situations. What use the animal makes of the mechanism is uncertain. It might be one method of localization in space and especially useful when, e.g. an eye-withdrawal reflex upsets the relationship between retina and surround, because eyecup position is not monitored by feedback from joint position receptors (Horridge and Sandeman, 1964; Wiersma and Oberjat, 1968). This joint appears in this respect to be different from all other known arthropod joints that are provided with appropriate sense cells. Finally, it may be noted that the rabbit's optokinetic system, which is similar in reflex features, is without this type of memory (Collewijn and van der Mark, 1972).

Information flow in the CNS

Ideally, one wants to know which particular input channels are involved in specific behavioral reactions. In some of the preceding chapters, several examples were presented where it was possible to trace with more or less confidence the pathways involved. As stated, when an interneuron with known input can be stimulated electrically, the pathway can be traced with more certainty. This is possible in only a few preparations, but even now other methods can be used to indicate the relationships. Examples of such an approach may be quoted from the crustacean visual system. Obviously the main difficulty involved is that any natural input affects very diverse interneurons, and one has to go through an elimination process to determine the main input channel. Inactivation of the parallel pathways as used by Kandel for this purpose (this volume) is not necessary under favorable conditions. One can, by knowing which central elements are specifically stimulated by a given input situation leading to a characteristic output, obtain weaker or stronger indications of the information flow in the CNS, even though all elements of the input-output chain have not been found. One such instance has been presented above, with relation to the seeing fibers and the antennal pointing reaction. In this case the chain is very incomplete, as it does not include any elements on the motor output side.

The neural chain of the reflexes, triggered by the angle at which light falls on the eye to the head-up and head-down optomotor fibers, is more strongly indicated. Here we find that light on front and back rim areas of the eye gives rise to reactions in identified sustaining and dimming fibers and causes appropriate reflex discharges in the motor fibers, representing a push-pull type of connectivity. Possibly these visual interneurons are directly and appropriately connected to the motor fibers. Further indication that the sustaining and/or dimming fibers are involved in the reflex discharges of these optomotor fibers comes from the following considerations: First, the sensory areas causing the optomotor reflex are essentially the same as those of the "rim" interneurons. Second, a synchronization of the discharge rate of the motor fibers with shadowing at a frequency of 5 to 10 per sec often occurs, and of all the fiber classes present in the optic nerve only sustaining and dimming fibers show continued short bursts during such stimulation. Since the visual interneurons apparently involved are but a few of the members of the two classes, the question arises what the functions of the others are. Likely, all are involved in more than one functional input-output relationship, and one could well be participation in the read-in and read-out systems involved in optokinetic memory.

For two major reflexes that can be visually elicited, the

input-output pathways are indicated even more certainly, because the visual area that triggers them is space constant. The escape reflex, mediated by the medial giant fibers, is triggered optically by quickly approaching objects. Because of the high thresholds of the giant fibers, it is difficult to obtain such optically triggered inputs. The reflex cannot be obtained from below in a crayfish in a transparent vessel, either in the normal or eye-down position of the animal. But in the latter situation, it can be obtained from both the dorsal and ventral halves of the upward pointing eye. This is exactly the same change in visual field as shown by the fast space-constant movement fiber. In the defense reflex, the animal takes up a characteristic position in which the claws and the head are raised. This position can be triggered when an axon with known location in the circumesophageal commissure is repetitively stimulated (Wiersma, 1952). This fiber is known to respond with firing to jittery motion in the visual field, such as finger movements (Wiersma and Mill, 1965), but that this reaction is space constant has not yet been proved. For the defense reflex, space constancy was shown by the methods described for the escape response. This indicates that the space-constant jittery movement fibers are the main input channels. Whereas electrical stimulation of the defense reflex fiber causes completely symmetrical output, during natural execution the animal orients towards the location of the stimulus also, presumably due to activity of parallel pathways signaling other aspects of the visual surround. Incomplete as this evidence is, it nevertheless shows that in some cases it is possible to approach the goal of determining information flow along the total pathway for rather complex behavioral events.

Present and future prospects for the study of neuronal behavior

It has been shown in this and other papers in this part, that one may, indeed, speak of the behavior of a neuron. This behavior, like that of the whole organism, is influenced by both present and past events and is therefore not readily predictable. However in many cases, interneuron behavior depends on fewer factors than that of the animal as a whole and therefore will be more amenable to analysis. Each animal possesses several populations of neurons that come to specific levels of activity only under definite sets of circumstances and these therefore provide good indications of what specific changes in the environment are important to the organism. One main problem still remains, how the overall reaction is determined in situations in which more than one group is activated.

From these considerations it follows that study of interneuronal behavior will lead to a better understanding of how total behavior evolves. As an example let us discuss the, as yet, incomplete facts concerning the attention mechanism of the lobster seeing fibers and its relation to the mechanism of the antennal pointing reaction. The pointing reaction may be regarded as behavior of the animal as a whole. Pointing does not arise from any specific center, whose inputs do not show an attention mechanism, but instead from a combination of inputs, each equipped with its own. Attention, then, is not a readily localized property but has a diffuse representation. Whether or not the additional integrative mechanism necessary for the pointing movement also has its own additional "attention" is hard to judge, although it would seem unnecessary. At any rate, the mechanism in single interneurons is more promising for detailed analysis of the underlying events than that of the whole animal. But before this analysis can be really fruitful, it will be necessary to obtain more information about the input connections of the seeing fibers in order to place accurately the location of the attention mechanism and of the events leading up to it. With regard to memory mechanisms, the same statement about diffuse locations can be made. Since the seeing fibers show short-term memories, the above argument also applies here. In addition, we have seen that for the optokinetic memory mechanisms more than one location is strongly indicated. The advantage of this system is that it is more consistent under experimental circumstances than that of the seeing fibers and that its output is easier to study. Again, the input channels are insufficiently known, and in both instances the prime question will be whether or not they can be resolved to the extent that their circuitry can be experimentally handled.

In general, two major difficulties are involved in studying the behavior of neurons. One is that their reactivity may be regulated by factors other than synaptic input, of which changes in chemical surround appear to be the most important. Such changes are likely to be gradual and should not be of major importance in the above systems when studied over short periods. Another difficulty is that communication between interneurons may depend partially or completely on input other than that caused by presynaptic spikes. A good example of such a system is the vertebrate retina, where all three neuronal elements involved in information transmission between the primary sense cells and the spike trains in the optic nerve fibers appear to communicate exclusively by electrotonic interactions. In this nerve net both feed-forward and feed-back aspects are present, with polarizing and depolarizing effects. Therefore, it will be difficult to decide, e.g. in the rabbit's retina, which ganglion cells are movement sensitive and which ones are "on"-center, "off"-surround from their anatomical connections with the presynaptic elements. When centrifugally provided information is present, as in the arthropod eye, this difficulty may be even greater, especially if such pathways end on more than one type of element. As far as information flow is concerned, such systems may have to remain black boxes until methods can be devised to deal with them and the underlying events thereby revealed. Nevertheless, studying their overall input-output relationships in terms of general input and spike discharge output will show what is being integrated. The study of such systems is therefore analogous to the study of the behavior of whole organisms. Note also that knowledge about which factors are important for the behavior of the diverse interneuronal classes may be of considerable aid in the design of behavioral experiments on the whole animal.

There has been a strong tendency to ignore the behavior of the neuron and emphasize the synaptic event level. I am convinced that this will not be successful in explaining behavior even though we may by these means be able to locate a certain aspect. For example, many cases of reflex habituation involve the synaptic transmission process between input fibers and a single postsynaptic cell (see Kandel for *Aplysia*, in this volume). But note here, that at other synapses such habituation appears to be completely absent, though the transmission processes seem very much alike. Certainly the reason for this difference is important from a neurophysiological point of view. However, it may not only take a long time to solve this problem but it is rather immaterial for behavior, as long as its consequences are understood. Aréchiga et al. (1973) found that habituation with the same characteristics as above is present in several crayfish interneurons. When the same habituating stimulus was presented to the common sensory area of interneurons with overlapping fields, different extents of habituated areas resulted. Realizing that such differences may depend on any of a number of factors, it is unrealistic to study all such subsystems in detail to provide for the final outcome. Also, as mentioned previously, synaptic connections differ so much from each other in function and properties that modelling at this level may be considered as a poor choice. Which relationships are present in any given case would not be known until each pathway was studied in great depth, and if one waited until this is done, no progress would be made in "neurological ethology." Certainly we should also be ill-advised to go the other way and neglect synaptology. However, in order to gain an understanding of what makes a central nervous system perform the functions it fulfills, and especially to gain insight into such problems as why certain cue stimuli are preferentially reacted to by certain species whereas they are replaced by different ones in closely related ones, the neuronal behavior approach is likely to provide answers more quickly.

One shortcoming in this general area that should be rather easy to remedy is lack of knowledge of the sum total of behavioral acts that a given species can perform. Such information is essential in order to be able to correlate the behavior of the neuron with that of the animal. This is true not only for invertebrates but also for most vertebrates. I hope I have shown that the neuronal behavioral approach is both interesting and intellectually challenging. I foresee an impressive growth for this field in the near future, as well as a long lifetime.

ACKNOWLEDGMENTS I am very grateful to Drs. H. Aréchiga, R. Hirsh, T. Yamaguchi, K. Yanagisawa, and B. York and the late Dr. Reddy, all of whom contributed to the research reported. My very special thanks are due to J. Roach for editorial comments. The research reported here has been supported by grants from the National Science Foundation and the National Institutes of Health, Public Health Service.

REFERENCES

ARÉCHIGA, H., B. BARRERA-MERA, and B. FUENTES-PARDO, 1973. Habituation of mechanoreceptive neurons of the crayfish. *J. Neurobiol.* (in press).

ARÉCHIGA, H., and C. A. G. WIERSMA, 1969a. The effect of motor activity on the reactivity of single visual units in the crayfish. *J. Neurobiol.* 1:53–69.

ARÉCHIGA, H., and C. A. G. WIERSMA, 1969b. Circadian rhythm of responsiveness in crayfish visual units. *J. Neurobiol.* 1:71–85.

BARNES, W. J. P., C. P. SPIRITO, and W. H. EVOY, 1972. Nervous control of walking in the crab. *Cardisoma guanhumi*. II. Role of resistance reflexes in walking. *Z. Vergl. Physiol.* 76:16–31.

BENNETT, M. V. L., and M. E. SPIRA, 1972. Synaptic control of electrotonic coupling between neurons. *Brain Res.* 37:294–300.

BUSH, B. M. H., 1965. Leg reflexes from chordotonal organs in the crab, *Carcinus maenas*. *Comp. Biochem. Physiol.* 15:567–587.

COLLEWIJN, H., and F. VAN DER MARK, 1972. Ocular stability in variable visual feedback conditions in the rabbit. *Brain Res.* 36:47–57.

DIJKGRAAF, S., 1956. Kompensatorische Augenstieldrehungen und ihre Auslösung bei der Languste (*Palinurus vulgaris*). *Z. Vergl. Physiol.* 38:491–520.

HORRIDGE, G. A., 1965. A direct response of the crab *Carcinus* to the movement of the sun. *Nature (London)* 207:1413–1414.

HORRIDGE, G. A., 1966. Optokinetic memory in the crab, *Carcinus*. *J. Exp. Biol.* 44:233–245.

HORRIDGE, G. A., 1968. Five types of memory in crab eye response. In *Physiological and Biochemical Aspects of Nervous Integration*, F. D. Carlson, ed., Englewood Cliffs, N.J.: Prentice-Hall, pp. 245–265.

HORRIDGE, G. A., and D. C. SANDEMAN, 1964. Nervous control of optokinetic responses in the crab *Carcinus*. *Proc. Roy. Soc. (London)* B161:216–246.

KANDEL, E. R., 1968. Dale's principle and the functional specificity of neurons. In *Cellular Pharmacology*, E. Coella, ed. Springfield, Ill.: Charles C Thomas, pp. 385–398.

KENNEDY, D., 1971. Crayfish interneurons. *The Physiologist* 14:5–30.

LINDBERG, R. G., 1955. Growth, population dynamics, and

field behavior in the spiny lobster, *Panulirus interruptus* (Randall). *Calif. Univ. Publ. Zool.* 59:157–247.

Mill, P. J., and D. A. Lowe, 1971. Transduction processes of movement and position sensitive cells in a crustacean limb proprioceptor. *Nature* (*London*) 229:206–208.

Shepheard, P. R. B., 1966. Optokinetic memory and the perception of movement by the crab, *Carcinus*. In *The Functional Organization of the Compound Eye*, C. G. Bernhard, ed. Oxford: Pergamon Press, pp. 543–557.

Spirito, C. P., W. H. Evoy, and W. J. P. Barnes, 1972. Nervous control of walking in the crab, *Cardisoma guanhumi*. I. Characteristics of resistance reflexes. *Z. Vergl. Physiol.* 76:1–15.

Whitear, M., 1962. The fine structure of crustacean proprioceptors. I. The chordotonal organs in the legs of the shore crab, *Carcinus maenas*. *Phil. Trans. Roy. Soc.* (*London*) B 245: 291–325.

Wiersma, C. A. G., 1952. Neurons of arthropods. *Cold Spring Harbor Symp. Quant. Biol.* 17:155–163.

Wiersma, C. A. G., 1958. On the functional connections of single units in the central nervous system of the crayfish, *Procambarus clarkii* (Girard). *J. Comp. Neurol.* 110:421–471.

Wiersma, C. A. G., 1959. Movement receptors in decapod crustacea. *J. Mar. Biol. Assoc., U.K.* 38:143–152.

Wiersma, C. A. G., and E. G. Boettiger, 1959. Unidirectional movement fibres from a proprioceptive organ of the crab, *Carcinus maenas*. *J. Exp. Biol.* 36:102–112.

Wiersma, C. A. G., and B. M. H. Bush, 1963. Functional neuronal connections between the thoracic and abdominal cords of the crayfish, *Procambarus clarkii* (Girard). *J. Comp. Neurol.* 121:207–235.

Wiersma, C. A. G., and G. M. Hughes, 1961. On the functional anatomy of neuronal units in the abdominal cord of the crayfish, *Procambarus clarkii* (Girard). *J. Comp. Neurol.* 116:209–228.

Wiersma, C. A. G., F. van der Mark, and L. Fiore, 1970. On the firing patterns of the "movement" receptors of the elastic organs of the crab, *Carcinus*. *Comp. Biochem. Physiol.* 34: 833–840.

Wiersma, C. A. G., and P. J. Mill, 1965. "Descending" neuronal units in the commissure of the crayfish central nervous system; and their integration of visual, tactile and proprioceptive stimuli. *J. Comp. Neurol.* 125:67–94.

Wiersma, C. A. G., and T. Oberjat, 1968. The selective responsiveness of various crayfish oculomotor fibers to sensory stimuli. *Comp. Biochem. Physiol.* 26:1–16.

Wiersma, C. A. G., and T. Yamaguchi, 1966. The neuronal components of the optic nerve of the crayfish as studied by single unit analysis. *J. Comp. Neurol.* 128:333–358.

Wiersma, C. A. G., and T. Yamaguchi, 1967. Integration of visual stimuli by the crayfish central nervous system. *J. Exp. Biol.* 47:409–431.

Wiersma, C. A. G., and K. Yanagisawa, 1971. On types of interneurons responding to visual stimulation present in the optic nerve of the rock lobster, *Panulirus interruptus*. *J. Neurobiol.* 2:291–309.

Wiersma, C. A. G., and B. York, 1972. Properties of the seeing fibers in the rock lobster: Field structure, habituation, attention, and distraction. *Vision Res.* 12:627–640.

Yoon, M., 1971. Reorganization of retinotectal projection following surgical operations on the optic tectum in goldfish. *Exp. Neurol.* 33:395–409.

Yoon, M., 1972. Reversibility of the reorganization of retinotectal projection in goldfish. *Exp. Neurol.* 35:565–577.

York, B., C. A. G. Wiersma, and K. Yanagisawa, 1972. Properties of the optokinetic motor fibres in the rock lobster: Build-up, flipback, afterdischarge and memory, shown by their firing patterns. *J. Exp. Biol.* 57:217–227.